STRENGTH TRAINING
FOR WOMEN

OLGA RÖNNBERG

STRENGTH TRAINING
FOR WOMEN

Training Programs, Food, and Motivation
for a Stronger, More Beautiful Body

Photographs by Andreas Lundberg
Translation by Gun Penhoat

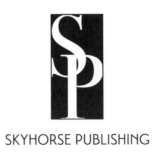

SKYHORSE PUBLISHING

Skyhorse Publishing books may be purchased in bulk at special discounts
for sales promotion, corporate gifts, fund-raising, or educational
purposes. Special editions can also be created to specifications. For
details, contact the Special Sales Department, Skyhorse Publishing, 307
West 36th Street, 11th Floor, New York, NY 10018 or
info@skyhorsepublishing.com.

Skyhorse® and Skyhorse Publishing® are registered trademarks of
Skyhorse Publishing, Inc.®, a Delaware corporation.

Visit our website at www.skyhorsepublishing.com.

10 9 8 7 6 5 4 3 2

Library of Congress Cataloging-in-Publication Data is available on file.

Cover photo credit: Andreas Lundberg

Print ISBN: 978-1-5107-0905-8
Ebook ISBN: 978-1-5107-0908-9

Printed in the United States of America

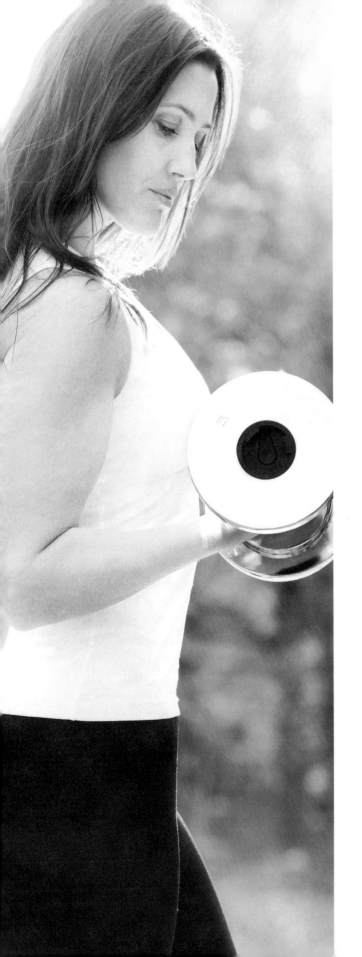

CONTENTS

You might already have a regular workout schedule and are now ready to tackle a bigger challenge. Perhaps you've worked out for several years but haven't been making much progress lately. Or maybe you've never weight trained before, but you'd like to learn how to do it correctly, from the start. Whatever your reason—this book is for you.

Myths often abound with regards to strength training, so allow me to dispel them. This book will show you that you won't become bulky; instead you'll develop a stronger and tighter body, cut a trimmer figure, and boost your self-confidence. Strength training is all about daring to be better and pushing oneself a little bit further.

Considering the many benefits you will reap, I sincerely hope you will get on board a strength training program even if you're unsure about giving it a try. Weight training strengthens the skeletal system, stimulates weight loss, decreases the risk of injury, increases stamina, and improves the quality of sleep. In other words, you'll have the energy to play with your kids; you can remain seated for longer periods of time without beginning to slouch; you'll be able to carry your grocery bags without your arms feeling like they're going to fall off; and you'll feel happier about your appearance. Is there anything wrong with these things?

My own interest in strength training began many years ago when I wanted to get back in shape after giving birth to my third child. Naturally, I was worried about developing bulky thighs and large biceps, but I closed my eyes, trusted the information I had read, and noticed my body's transformation—and I fell in love. The love is still going strong to this day; I yearn for my dumbbells every morning. Even now, it's such a joy to grab a pair of heavy weights and think of how far I've come with the help of strength training. It's still a special feeling to walk into a gym and take in the smell of metal—weight training doesn't just change you physically, it enables you to evolve mentally as well. You push, you hold, you wring every last ounce of energy from your muscles—and you'll feel like a winner.

So, welcome to the exciting world of strength training! I promise you results you could once only dream of. That is on the condition, of course, that you don't skip any of these steps or break from the program's routines. Make the best of what you have, push yourself hard, and enjoy your success!

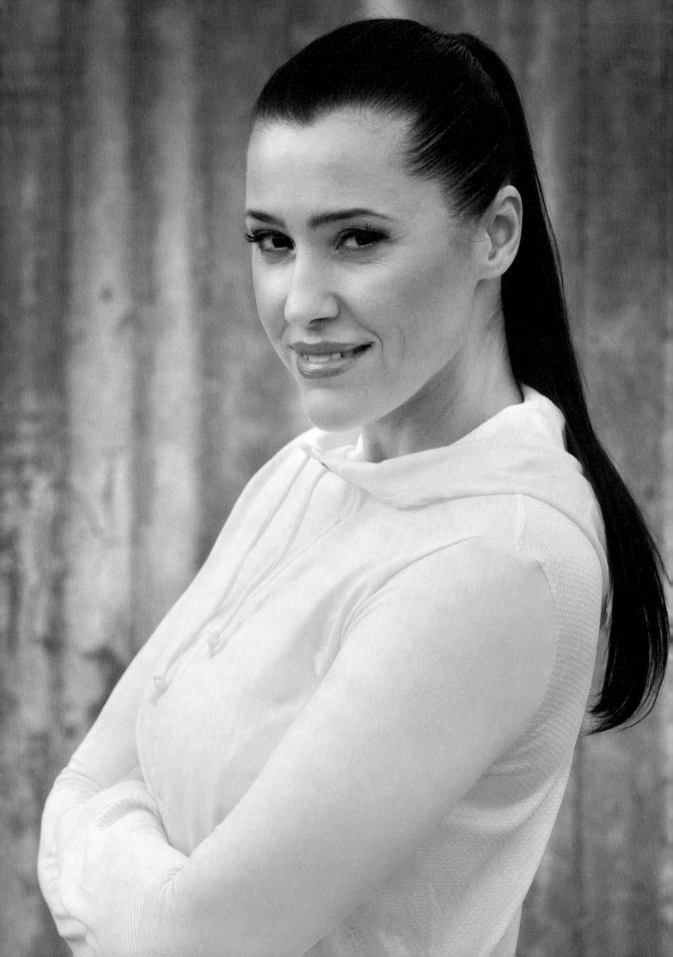

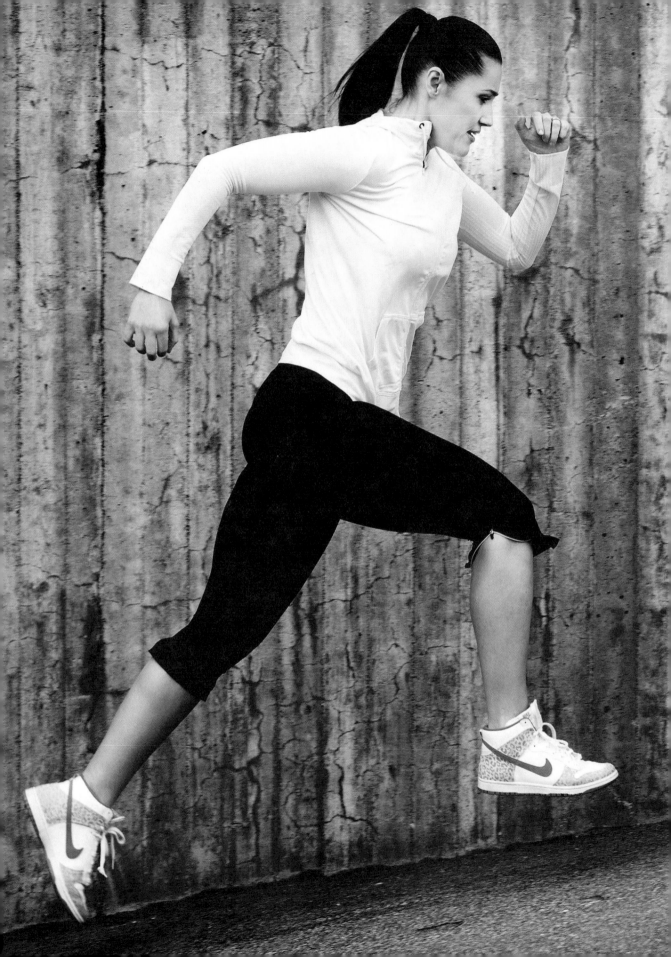

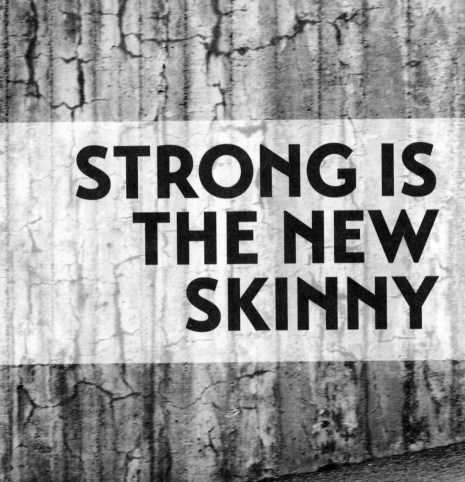

Many of us are fed up with the fuss of complicated food and training regimens. We want something that works for us over the long haul as well as in the here and now of everyday life. We are tired of deprivation diets, elaborate workout routines, and of feeling hungry while not achieving the goals we set for ourselves.

To that end, a number of us have discovered strength training. We want to develop more muscles, and we want to feel strong. Muscles have become a status symbol because they're physical proof that a person is disciplined and works hard for what he or she wants. A skinny body is no longer a desirable goal; today, we want to show off our "guns" and wear tight-fitting jeans. Strong has become the new skinny, and it's all for the better! Not only does strength training strengthen your muscles, it also improves your posture, increases your metabolism, and rallies your mental health. It staves off injuries and reduces the general wear and tear on your body. In short, you will become fitter and healthier in your daily life.

Why do we need a book about strength training, especially one catered to women? Aren't women able to work out like men? Do we even need to strength train? Why can't we just go running instead? Don't you become brawny the moment you start lifting weights? There is a slew of misinformation about strength training out there, especially regarding weight training for women. How often do I hear the words, "I want a toned body, not bulky muscles!"

Ask any man who lifts weights how easy it is to build muscle mass, and he'll most likely answer, "It's difficult," or "It takes a long time." Furthermore, the hormonal makeup of women makes it even more challenging for us to build large muscles. Our levels of testosterone are significantly lower than men's, so only years of heavy, intense training can make us look anything like a man in the muscles department.

It's vital for women to do regular weight training since we often work at sedentary jobs, where we are seated most of the time. Many of us also go through pregnancy and birth, which puts great strain on our bodies. Hence the health benefits of strength training: it makes the body stronger from the inside out, muscles and bones become more powerful, and the entire body becomes healthier and more beautiful.

What's more, the earlier you start working out in life, the better. We are at our physical peak around the age of twenty-five, and our natural physical decline typically begins at age forty.

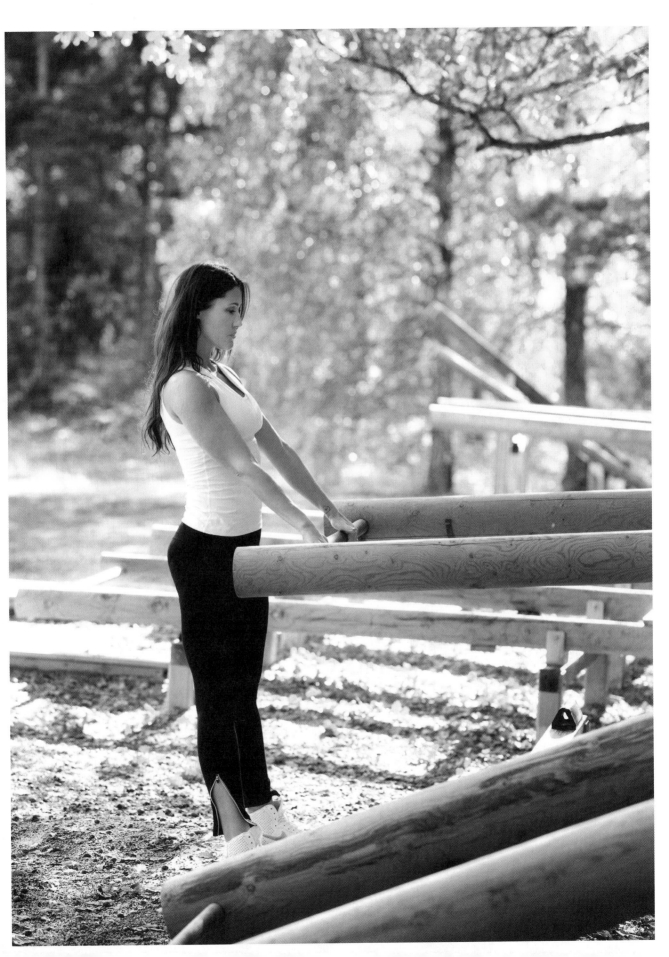

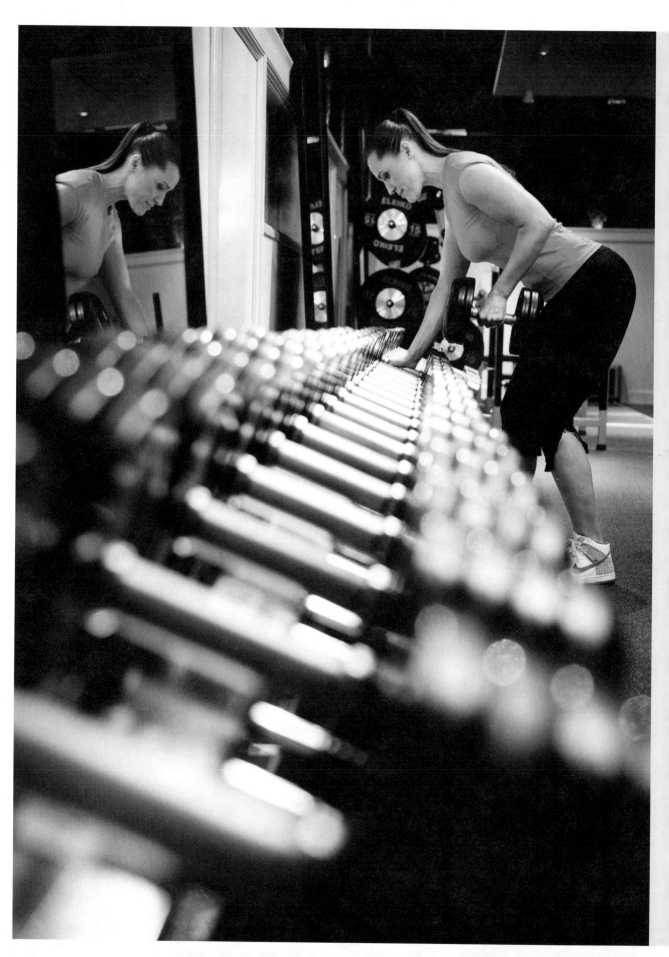

When muscle mass starts to decrease and fat stores accumulate, many women get in touch with me to ask me if it's too late to do anything, and I'm only too happy to report that it's still possible to become fit! Not only am I living proof of this, I'm also able to point to my own clients' results—women who are fully engaged in midlife, with all that this entails. Women who try to become fit by focusing on weight loss, whether through fad diets, excess exercise, or both, often feel increased levels of stress. They feel they've made bad nutritional choices, and they suffer from disrupted sleep patterns, impaired immunity, slower metabolism, and hormonal disturbances—all things that can get in the way of successful weight loss or weight maintenance. On the other hand, strength training makes it easier to become fit and trim in a sustainable and healthy way. And it's never too late to start—you can build muscles at any age, you can lose weight at any age, and you can become stronger and more energetic, whether you are twenty-five, forty, or seventy years old. But you have to put in the work. Good outcomes require input in the form of physical activity and proper nutrition. This is not something you can indulge in sporadically—you need to make a conscious effort and focus on every workout and meal. You will train more intensely than you have ever done before; you will sweat and feel out of breath. You won't be lifting a pair of dumbbells while thinking about what you're going to fix for dinner later; no, you will work out with a purpose: to change how you look and feel. To do this you will need to set aside some time. And your diet might need to be modified or changed completely, depending on where you are at today.

In this book, I will cheer you on to become stronger than you ever thought possible. The book consists of three steps—building, fine-tuning, and burning. The only thing you need to do is follow the program to the letter.

Since building a strong and beautiful body is as much about nutrition as it is about working out, there is a dietary part to each step, which includes an ingredient list as well as recipes, so you know what to do and how to go about eating healthier.

Keep in mind that the focus of this book is not on weight loss per se but on building muscle and losing fat, which is an effective strategy to achieve permanent weight loss.

BEFORE YOU BEGIN

I believe that fitness is more of a mental challenge than a physical one. Why? Because everything starts in your mind. If you want something enough, you'll be sure to make it happen.

It needs to be crystal clear to you that the outcome will depend entirely on your effort and work. You get returns based on what you put into it, so if you train well, eat properly, and follow the program exactly, I guarantee that you will succeed. Perform your workout at the time of day when you feel most energetic to make it easier and more enjoyable.

Find a buddy who shares the same goals as you. Go through the program together and follow the same diet. The two of you can cheer each other on if the going gets tough.

Think about your motive for taking up this training. What is the reason you want to start this program? Is it to become stronger? Is it to feel better or to look more attractive? Whatever reasons you have, they must be your own; they can't be your neighbor's, your friend's, or your spouse's. It's difficult to keep yourself inspired day after day—that's entirely normal—but if you don't lose sight of the reasons for doing what you're doing, it will make things far more agreeable, I promise!

Finally: Make your commitment a priority, and take it seriously. This is about you, your health, and your well-being. You want to feel good in your own skin. This is time well spent.

GOALS AND DEADLINES

It's important to know where you're heading and what your end goal is. It needs to be realistic and to take into account your current state of health. Reaching your goal could be either more challenging or easier than you think. We are not going to follow any magical or miracle method published in some magazine, so remember to set attainable objectives. You haven't done anything wrong if you come to realize that your goal is not achievable in the time frame you have set for yourself. Even if you're doing everything right, you might have set your sights a little too high. So, why not set up partial goals? They will enable you to easily check if you're on the right track. If you find yourself off course, you can make the necessary adjustments in a timely way.

You can't set a goal without having a deadline, i.e., when your goal should be reached. Personally, I like it when people breathe down my neck—I feel pressed for time and focused. So, I have already scheduled a deadline for you: mark a day on your calendar six months ahead from today's date. That will give you plenty of time to establish good habits, and your workouts will have had time to take effect.

FOOD AND TRAINING LOG

Keeping a food and exercise log is essential! If you think it's boring and unnecessary, remember that all elite athletes keep track of every one of their training opportunities. There is a good reason for this: it enables you to follow the path toward your goals. If your earlier training session wasn't that great, you can simply check your log entry and think about how it could be improved upon.

The food log can be used as a tool to monitor what and how much you eat. Maybe you'll uncover a pattern that you can tweak for the better. Many are surprised to see how little real food they eat and how much junk food they consume in a single day.

At the end of this book, you'll find an example of how a food and training log can be set up. Try to fill it out and analyze your results. Perhaps you'll be surprised at what you actually eat in a day or be amazed at how quickly you're building strength from the get-go.

TOOLS

This program's tools include dumbbells, a stability ball, a weight bench, and a barbell.

It doesn't matter if you work out at home or in a gym; that's your choice. You won't be able to use the excuse of not having time to go to the gym because you can also work out in your living room. If you prefer to work out at home, that's okay, but you must use weights that enable you to complete five reps—they must be heavy enough to challenge your strength. Probably the biggest downside to working out at home is that you must invest in proper equipment. Some don't believe this, and they think that 11- to 22-pound weights (5–10 kg) are more than adequate for the job. That might be true for the short term, but your workout will quickly become ineffective if the weight becomes too light for you. Proper weights are a necessary tool to getting good results. Typically, women have less upper-body strength and more lower-body strength, so if you wish to combine gym and home workout sessions, it would be smart to train your upper body at home, and your lower body at the gym where you'll have access to heavier weights.

If you have a choice between using free weights (such as dumbbells and barbells) and machines, always opt for the free weights. When you're stuck in the single position with a machine, there's no way to balance and stabilize your body in a natural way as you would if you were using free weights. Machine exercises are too isolating and are designed to focus on only one muscle/muscle group at a time. However, if you use free weights you'll be working the muscle from different angles and also roping in assistance from other muscles while you're at it.

TRAINING CLASSES

If you peek into an aerobics class, you won't notice many well-trained women (read: with muscles) in there. Don't get me wrong—I'm all for moving about, but I believe in getting results from a workout and having a goal in mind. If you're looking for solid gains in strength, you won't get it from participating in an aerobics class; not even strength training classes will do this for you. There are too many repetitions per exercise and the tempo is too quick, which means you don't have enough time to stretch the muscle to its fullest, and consequently your form will suffer. Form tops the list when it comes to strength training. You don't want to get injured! If you're a beginner, a training class might help you at first, but after a while you'll hit a plateau (read more about plateaus on page 28), and your progress will slow down or stall altogether.

When you work out using your own program, you're able to follow your own particular developing strength. You can adjust your exercise routine to fit your capabilities with respect to rest periods, pace, and the amount of weight you need to use. This makes for optimal training because it is tailored to your specific needs.

MEASURE YOUR PROGRESS!

Take your "before" pictures now! Timeline photos are a very motivating way to track your progress. Muscles take up less space than fat, so your bathroom scale won't be a useful tool for measuring results when you're strength training.

Another way of taking stock is to record how everything feels. What do you see when you look in the mirror, and what do others say? It's easy to become blind to our own reflection because we see ourselves every day, so trust that others will see what you are unable to.

THE BENEFITS OF STRENGTH TRAINING

There are many ways in which strength training affects the body. I have listed some of its positive effects so you don't forget why it's important to keep up with your workouts.

SHORTER STRENGTH-TRAINING WORKOUTS MAKE A BIG IMPACT

You don't need to work out for hours at a time, because it's not important how long you exercise, it's important how *smart* you exercise. That's what result-oriented training is all about. If you work out for longer than an hour, your performance will decline and you'll be able to lift less and less.

STRENGTH TRAINING'S POSITIVE EFFECTS ON THE BODY

Not many know or think about strength training's positive effects on the body. How about the following? Strength training

- increases muscular strength
- increases cardiovascular endurance
- increases blood circulation
- increases fat burning (up to 48 hours after a workout)
- increases maximal oxygen uptake (VO_2 max)
- lowers blood pressure
- improves metabolism
- strengthens the skeleton
- improves sleep
- reduces the risk for cardiovascular disease

You might think you have all these benefits with cardiovascular training alone. However, you won't improve your posture or build a stronger back and shoulders by running; you won't strengthen your abdominal muscles by walking; and you won't increase your amount of fast-twitch muscle fibers through Nordic walking. Muscle strength can't be acquired solely through aerobic training. On the other hand, strength training can help you become a better runner, thus preventing you from sustaining running-related injuries.

STRENGTH TRAINING MAKES FOR EFFICIENT FAT BURNING

The key to weight loss is a faster metabolism. While both strength training and cardio training will give your metabolic rate a boost, it's more readily achieved through strength training. *Intensity* is the key word here. If you push your body to work hard, it will release performance-enhancing hormones in order to survive. When this is done in a consistent manner, these hormones will have a positive effect on your metabolism. With strength training, you'll become a more efficient fat burner. Of course, aerobic activity such as running or spinning is healthy for you, but as your body quickly adapts to the workload, you'll have to keep ramping up the intensity and length of your workouts to maintain your metabolic rate. Who has time for this?

Strength training triggers a boost of energy after-burn that can last up to 48 hours after a workout. At this point, additional muscle cells begin to grow, which in turn increases your muscle mass as well as your basal metabolism (read more about this on p. 20).

COMMON MISCONCEPTIONS ABOUT STRENGTH TRAINING

There are lots of myths about strength training out there, and I will deal with a few of the most common ones. How on earth did these come about?

LONG OR BULKY MUSCLES

A common misconception about weight training is that working with small weights produces long slim muscles, while lifting heavy weights produces large, bulky muscles. A muscle can only become larger or smaller. Regardless of how you work out, you can't choose to make your biceps bulky or long and slim. This is as unrealistic as attempting to change your height—it doesn't work.

YOU WILL NOT BECOME RIPPED OVERNIGHT

To build muscle you need testosterone; we women typically have very low levels of this hormone. The female bodybuilders you see in pictures train strenuously for many years. In addition, a certain genetic predisposition is needed for this body type, and occasionally illegal supplements and drugs are taken in order to achieve that look. Adding a lot of muscle mass requires a lot of energy—i.e., a lot of food. Keep in mind that I have seldom seen women overeat—it's usually the opposite—so believe me when I tell you that you will not become a hulk of muscle overnight. If you still think you carry too much muscle mass, decrease the amount of weight you are lifting.

MY MUSCLES WILL TURN TO FAT IF I STOP WORKING OUT

This is like saying my right hand will turn into my right foot. Fat and muscle are two separate body tissues, so if you eat more and train less, what will happen is your muscles will shrink in size, and you might increase your fat stores. Muscle tissue burns fat while fat tissue stores extra energy. So why would you want to stop working out?

GET TO KNOW YOUR BODY

We all have different genetic set points, so even if we follow an identical workout program we will still end up looking different and get a variety of results. Even if your level of body fat is low, you still might not see your midsection's six-pack—and that's just one example. This is why I warn against comparing your body to others. Life isn't fair. The best you can do is to always, always, always use your own base condition and abilities as a starting point. If you compare yourself to others, you'll have trouble judging your own progress objectively.

YOUR MUSCLES

It's important to be aware of what you are training and which muscles you are trying to affect with each different type of exercise. Your body has about 640 muscles. I won't be tackling all of them in these workout programs, but I will be concentrating on the large muscle groups from where you draw your everyday strength: back, glutes, legs, and chest. The large muscle groups use up a lot of energy and support both your posture and various physical movements in order to help you carry your body with pride.

MUSCLE ACHES

Do you have to push yourself until your muscles ache after each workout? If you never feel muscles soreness, is your workout ineffective? There is no single answer as to why muscles ache. Sore muscles are, more than anything, a gauge of how fit or unfit a person is. It's common to feel achy when switching up exercises, working out with heavier weights, or upping the intensity of a workout. Not feeling sore doesn't mean your workout is useless, however. Remember that we are all unique, even in this instance.

BASAL METABOLIC RATE (BMR)

The Basal Metabolic Rate, or BMR, indicates how much energy is needed for basic existence and taking care of bodily functions while you're at rest. Quite a lot of energy is needed just to keep the body going—the internal organs go through their processes, the heart beats, the brain thinks, food is digested, we perspire and breathe, and so on. BMR varies from person to person and is partially steered by genetic material. It affects, among other things, how efficiently the body is at digesting food, storing it, and using it for fuel. BMR is typically higher in men than in women, since women tend to have a higher percentage of body fat. A person's BMR can be calculated using his or her gender, age, height, and weight. You can read more about how to calculate your BMR on page 41.

WHAT IS YOUR BODY TYPE?

We often talk about four distinct body types, but of course we're all more or less a combination of these different types. Check the list below to see what type best fits to you.

Hourglass: The waist is smaller than the upper and lower body. Fat distribution is even; you can store and lose fat quite easily. You have good ability to build muscle.

Pear: The lower body is proportionally larger than the upper body, with heavy thighs and calves. The trunk and upper body muscles are not especially strong. You have a good ability to build muscles.

Apple: This is a round body shape, largest circumference being across the belly. Muscles in your upper body are not that strong; you can store fat easily but have difficulty losing it.

Rectangle: Chest, waist, and hips are of equal width. You find it difficult to build muscles and can sometimes store fat around the belly. You probably have quite good cardiovascular endurance but have insignificant muscle mass.

How our body appears, and how it is affected by exercise and nutrition, are highly unique to each individual. Keep in mind that your results are only dependent on about thirty to forty percent of your genetic heritage; the rest is up to you. I say *only* because you have a direct impact on how you work out, on what you choose to do, and on how you eat. With strength training, you can sculpt your body as you wish—wide shoulders and a broad back will make your waist appear smaller, and if your hips are wider than your shoulders you will become proportionally balanced if you focus on working up your shoulders. Isn't that great? Best of all: intensity trumps genes. The harder you work out, the less genes matter.

HORMONES

When you're thirty years old, you're still pretty near the top of your natural abilities in terms of strength and general fitness. You're well-coordinated, have good balance, and a ready supply of energy. Perhaps you've had your first child and have been in the workforce for a few years. Have you noticed that it isn't as easy to lose weight as it was when you were in your twenties? Maybe you're heading toward your forties. If you have been mostly sedentary, now is the time you will start to feel the effects of being inactive—and it will begin to show, too. And if you have been active, you might begin to notice that you need longer to recuperate between workouts and that you need your sleep.

There could be a lot of reasons for this, not just whether you've kept up on your workouts or not. Hormones, pregnancy, a sedentary work environment, thyroid problems, stress, medications, or bad nutritional habits can all make your body feel like it isn't "running" as well as it once did. All these factors can hamper your ability to achieve results. Many women require another strategy than just working out and following a special diet.

METABOLISM AND MUSCLE MASS

There are some things we need to take into consideration when we talk about "female" fat burning. Some of us have a long past of dysfunctional eating behavior, such as not eating enough food (too few calories), yo-yo dieting, eating too much sugar, and even ingesting too little protein and healthy fat. Metabolism is often slowed down by insufficient food, long and strenuous aerobic workouts, and not training with weights (weight training has shown to have a positive effect on metabolism). But don't despair! We can improve your body's constitution if we grab hold of it now. Eat more (including additional protein), eat regularly, strength train with weights, avoid overly long aerobic workouts, avoid eating simple carbohydrates, and reduce your levels of stress. Eat better, not less. Do short, intense training sessions rather than long, drawn-out workouts.

You could lose up to half your body's total muscle mass from your twenties up to your nineties. There are many reasons for this, but bad nutrition and inactivity are major culprits. After fifty years of age you're also losing muscle mass at a faster rate, about one to two percent per year. Muscle mass is the main determinant of how much energy you expend while you're at rest. Compare 2¼ lbs (1kg = 1,000g) of fat, which burns 4 kcal/day, to 2¼ lbs of muscle, which incinerates approximately 70 kcal/day. For many women, this is the difference between being reasonably fit and being overweight. You don't want to lose any muscles! When you lose muscle mass, your metabolism slows down. To build muscles, you have to challenge them continuously to make them stronger. A surefire way to do this is to begin lifting weights.

MY STRENGTH-TRAINING PRINCIPLES

It's good to know what to do and how to think when you start out with your training. I'm going to mention a few principles that you should always be mindful of when you're working out to ensure faster and better results.

PROGRESSIVE OVERLOAD

The body quickly adapts to current conditions, even when working out. This is both good and bad.

To avoid stagnating, it's important to keep progress in mind when we work out. This can mean moving on to heavier weights, increasing the amount of sets or repetitions, or switching out some exercises for different or more challenging variations.

BE SPECIFIC

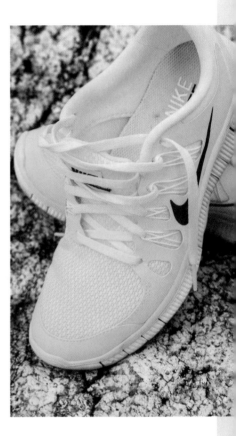

You are good at what you do! If you want more defined muscles but you're dancing in a Zumba class, what do you think is going to happen? I have nothing against Zumba, but do you think you can achieve what you want by dancing? What I'm trying to say is that you have to match your workout to your ultimate goal. If you want to master pushups, you have to work your chest, core, and arms. If you want to run faster in a race, train for that. You want a bigger glutes? You guessed it—train for that. Consider attending a Zumba class as your reward and not your main workout. *Kill your darlings!*

FREQUENCY

Here, I'm referring to how often you should work out. If you want to get good at something or achieve a goal, you must practice often and regularly. Use a schedule to ink in a certain amount of recurring workouts per week. Follow it on a regular basis and for longer uninterrupted periods of time.

INTENSITY

When we talk about workouts, intensity refers to performing an exercise with enough intensity that it becomes extremely difficult to finish—the last three repetitions should be close to the maximum effort you can manage.If you are strength training or running intervals, it's the push to muscle failure. Keep the workout lively and the intensity high. Once you're confident about proper form, increase the difficulty. Don't sit when you can stand, use free weights rather than machines, and perform basic moves instead of isolation exercises. The objective is to reach your goal quickly and not to run for a long time, right?

RECOVERY—REST AND SLEEP

"You grow when you sleep" is a common saying in the world of fitness. The body uses its time at rest to refill its energy stores and to build muscles. Training is stressful for the body; even if physical activity is good for the hormonal system, it's still important not to overdo things. Signs that you are over-training can include: stalled progress, injuries that take a long time to heal, and feeling low or depressed. What you eat is an important factor in good recovery, as is adequate rest. Be mindful of your body's signals, decrease your levels of stress, and make sure you get enough sleep.

PERIODIZATION

You shouldn't train too hard or too intensely for long periods. Check your goals—if you want to get stronger, your workouts should be geared for that; if you want to peel off layers of fat but retain as much muscle mass as possible, they should be tuned differently; if you want your muscles to grow, yet another workout will do the trick. It's quite common to find runners doing more strength training in the fall and winter, while focusing on running through spring and summer. Many who focus on muscle growth in the winter months will get "cut" in the spring—i.e., they will trim subcutaneous fat to achieve more defined and visible muscles tone.

A FEW IMPORTANT TERMS TO BECOME FAMILIAR WITH

- **Repetitions (or reps):** A completed exercise, performed from start to finish. The amount of reps depends on your training goal.

- **Set:** An amount of repetitions that are performed continuously without rest in between. The amount of sets depends on your training goal.
- **Supersets:** Two exercises performed one after the other with no rest in between. They're a great way of shocking the muscle and increasing training volume over a short time.
- **Circuit training:** Several exercises done one after the other without any rest in between.
- **Tempo:** The rate at which you move the weights up and down.
- **Rest:** Rest period between sets.

ADJUST THE NUMBER OF REPETITIONS TO FIT YOUR GOAL

The amount of repetitions you do per set will depend on your specific goals; below, you can see how certain amounts of repetitions will affect your development.

- Strength development, muscle growth: 1–6 repetitions
- Muscle growth, strength development: 6–15 repetitions

Naturally, muscle growth is affected no matter how many repetitions you perform, but there are more or less optimal ways in which you can reach these goals.

AEROBIC TRAINING

Aerobic training—or cardio training, as I will refer to it from here on—improves the body's capacity to use oxygen, strengthens the heart, affects metabolism and mood, lowers blood pressure, strengthens the immune system, and stabilizes blood sugar. You'll derive a lot of health benefits by engaging in it.

Cardio training is convenient since it doesn't require a lot of planning—you just put on a pair of sneakers, and you're on your way. It's easy to do, even when you're traveling. Cardio burns fat, too, if done the right way.

It can be done inside or outside, and on a treadmill, an elliptical, a bike, a rowing machine, or a step machine. Swimming is excellent exercise, too. When you train on cardio machines, it is extremely important that you do not lean on them for support. If you have a tendency to do this, decrease your speed. If you walk outside, a good way to stay motivated is to use a pedometer.

It doesn't matter at what time of the day you do your cardio training; the best time is whenever you are able to do it. Some people prefer mornings while others have more energy in the evening. I like to work out in the morning because it has positive psychological side effects. Morning workouts make you want to continue to do well by eating right the rest of the day, and you have more incentive to stick with it. However, do what suits you best. Have you ever wondered if cardio on an empty stomach is more effective than, say, cardio on your lunch break or in the evening? Well, it really doesn't matter that much in the grand scheme of things. Cardio training while fasting doesn't burn that many more calories than training at any other time, so I wouldn't worry about it.

Many use cardio training as a primary tool for weight loss, and as a result they work out incorrectly. Cardio training every day, and over longer periods of time, tends to have negative effects on your body, such as putting too much strain on your joints. Frequent, repetitive moments produce stress over time. This combined with insufficient recovery can lead to injuries, over-training, and a lowered immune system response. If your body is pear-shaped or apple-shaped and your goal is to lose weight with cardio exercise alone, what will you end up looking like? Like a somewhat smaller pear or apple, but still a pear and still an apple. However, as mentioned earlier, with strength training you can sculpt your body to your liking. As with most things, there are more or less efficient ways of going about it. My aim is to show you that the fastest and most effective way to reach your goal is to use a combination of cardio and strength training. Also, I'm going to separate cardio training into two levels: low intensity and high intensity exercise.

LOW INTENSITY CARDIO EXERCISE

Low intensity cardio workouts can be used very effectively together with strength training. This type of exercise burns calories without negatively impacting your recovery from a strength workout. Low intensity cardio can be performed before as well as after strength workouts, as you save your energy for the strength you'll need to lift weights.

Low intensity cardio exercise is stress-free and gentle on your joints, and it keeps muscles healthy. However, it might also be boring and more time-consuming, since workouts typically take about 60 to 90 minutes. Fat is used as your main source of fuel. Your target heart rate should be 60 to 65 percent of your maximum heart rate, which you can calculate by subtracting your age from 226, then multiplying the result by 0.65. If you are forty years old, this would be the calculation:

$$226 - 40 \times 0.65 = 120.9$$

Or, to put it simply: you should be able to keep a conversation going without becoming winded.

HIGH INTENSITY CARDIO EXERCISE

There are different types of high intensity cardio, my preference being HIIT (High Intensity Interval Training). HIIT training means alternating between bursts of high intensity activity, followed by rest periods. One example is running 110 yards (100 m) at your maximum, all-out effort, then coming back to the starting line at a slower pace, and repeating this sequence several times.

The principal argument in favor of HIIT cardio is that it affects the body's hormonal system in the same way as weight lifting. Anabolic hormones such as testosterone and the growth hormone, which are key to building and preserving muscle mass, can increase substantially by practicing HIIT.

HIIT exercise can also increase the body's ability to burn fat by boosting its metabolism.

The point to interval training is that you burn calories both during and after the workout, thanks to the so called "after-burn effect" or EPOC (excess post-exercise oxygen consumption), whose benefits include cell repair, hormone balance control, replenishment of energy stores, and muscle growth. All this means that you're still burning energy fairly long after the end of your workout.

The target heart rate should be around 85 to 90 percent of your maximum heart rate. If you don't have a heart rate monitor, make sure that you're properly winded and can only speak with some effort, that you've got a good sweat going, and that you can start to feel a touch of lactic acid buildup in your legs.

WHAT'S THE BEST FIT FOR YOU?

The very best routine will consist of a combination of high and low intensity cardio exercises. Since you can only perform HIIT a few times per week for it to be effective as a fat-burner, you'll need to add in some low intensity variations. I will show you how to do this within each training program. With each step, your cardio training requirements will vary, as will your calorie requirements.

PLATEAUS

You might notice that your results start to level off over a period of time, both in terms of weight and in measurements. This means that you've hit a plateau. For me, a plateau is when you've stopped seeing any progress in measurements and weight for about three weeks. You can end up there even if you've done everything by the book and slavishly followed both diet and workouts. It's easy to start obsessing and worrying about having done something wrong, which is where you run the risk of wanting to give up and try something else, whether it is another diet or workout program. Don't give up; just think of it as part of the process. The body does change, even if you can't measure it or see it with the naked eye.

Here are my tips on what to do to bust a plateau:

- Be especially careful with your calorie intake. Double-check that you're doing things right and that your arithmetic is correct.
- Bump up your training with one extra cardio workout (this is especially important in the third step).

- How intense are your cardio workouts? Do you really exert yourself, or have you stopped challenging yourself?

- Do you experience fluid retention even if you're not menstruating and you're not ovulating? If so, take a rest day to de-stress.

- Increase your food intake by 200 to 300 extra calories for a few days. Sometimes you have to shock the system, especially if your body is starting to adapt to the same calorie intake.

- Add a few extra sets of some special exercises—go for dead lifts, squats, and rowing. Use the large muscle groups that burn a lot of energy.

- Change your type of cardio. If you walk, bike. If you run on a treadmill, get on the elliptical machine.

- Are you lifting weights that are heavy enough? Are you really going full out and giving it your all?

If none of my tips above help, relax and continue your routine. Things will change, I promise.

THE IMPORTANCE OF KEEPING A TRAINING LOG

If you're serious about your training, I advise you to start a training log to keep track of your progress. It'll give you a good overview on your developing strength, and it can even work as a good motivator. Don't rely on your memory to remember the amount of weight you lifted four or five weeks ago; it's impossible!

On page 142, I show an example of how a training log might look. Fill it out for a day and see if this is something that could work for you.

Let's go!

I hope you've learned that while intensity is essential, form must not be sacrificed. Don't forget that our bodies have different capacities for change, but you can still rebuild your body through strength training. As you go along, you'll gain self-confidence and improve your well-being.

Now that your knowledge has broadened a bit, and you understand how this book is laid out as well as the purpose behind the steps, it's time to look at how and what you should eat in order to achieve your desired outcome.

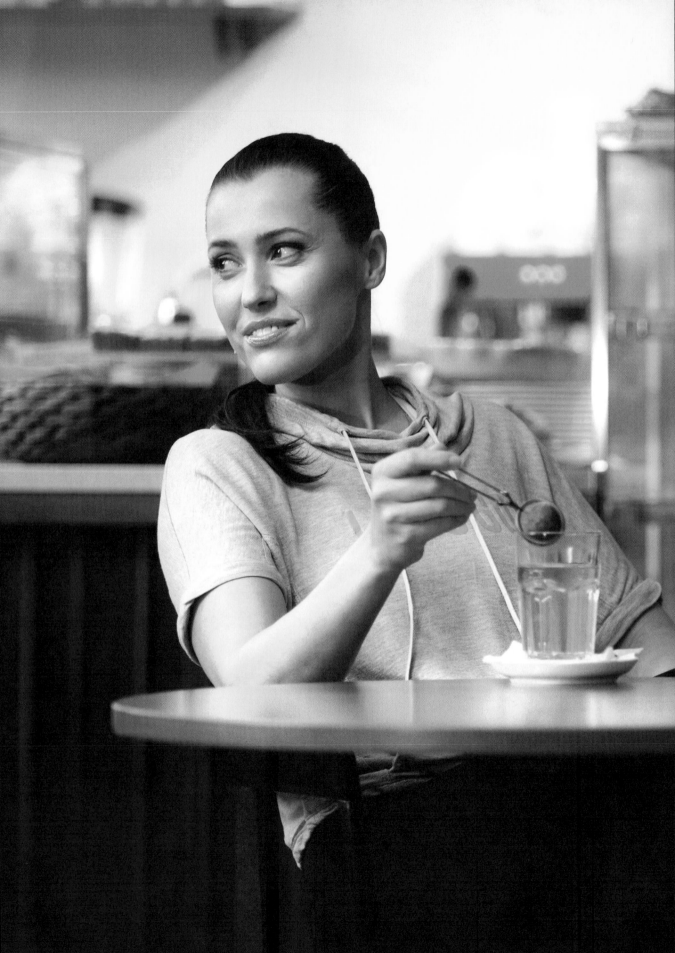

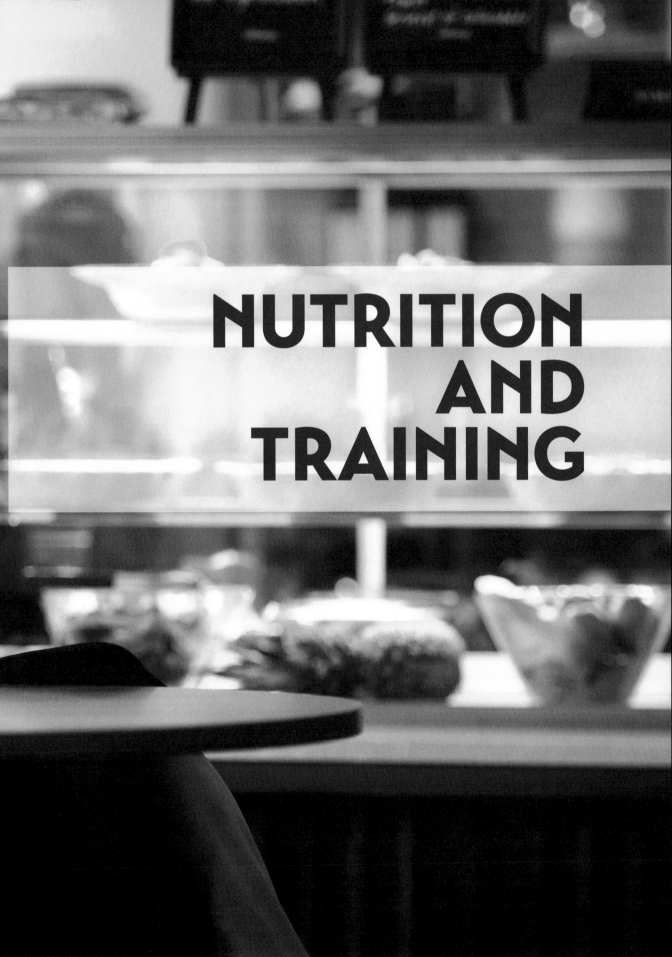

NUTRITION AND TRAINING

Nutrition has become a hot topic in the media, at home, and at work—everybody has his or her own opinion on how to eat right. For me, food is all about taking in the right kind of fuel at the right time. Good fuel is connected to how I run my life. I train, I work, I take care of my home and my kids. All this requires energy. I always make sure to eat enough so I can deal with my day without collapsing from exhaustion in the middle of it.

Training is not the only important component to achieving results; nutrition plays an equally important role. And, without a doubt, food is the aspect most of us have trouble with. No surprise—new findings are presented almost daily with new books, new diets, and up-to-the-minute research that contradict each other, all of which make things more confusing and bewildering. What's the right way to go about this? Should we weigh our food? Count calories? I believe in eating as cleanly as possible (by which I refer to consuming food without additives), avoiding simple and fast-acting carbohydrates, eating plenty of vegetables and protein, and including good carbohydrates and healthy fats.

Keep in mind that your particular training goals should dictate your intake of energy. If you're focusing on building muscle you'll need to eat a certain amount of food; however, if you want to trim fat you'll have different caloric requirements. If you wish to become a better athlete and run faster around the track, you'll need to follow a diet with that goal in mind. Many women want to be too many things at once, but their calorie intake is often too low, so, predictably, they make no headway. My advice is to concentrate on one goal for a period of time to allow your body to become accustomed to a set amount of calories, which will enable you to gauge your progress more accurately.

To reach your goals, you'll need to take stock of your current habits. We are what we do every day. Becoming fitter after living a sedentary life will require an overhaul of one's routines. This is true even with food, because in order to stay the course you have to engage in certain behaviors. For example, you'll need to draw up a meal plan and brown-bag your food wherever you go. It might seem unrealistic now, not to mention dorky, but wait and see—you'll soon be caught up in the spirit of it!

All food contains a variety of nutrients. I will show you the benefits of each type of food and teach you how to calculate your calorie requirements and adjust them to suit your training. I will also list the ingredients I keep in my pantry, explain the merits of keeping a food journal, and share my favorite recipes. But, let's start with the basics—what is food?

PROTEIN

After looking through hundreds of food journals, I know many women don't eat enough protein. Many of us believe that high levels of protein bring about large muscles and that eating lettuce is a plan for losing weight. Sorry—you couldn't be more mistaken.

Protein is the most important nutrient for both building muscles and weight loss. Protein keeps you satiated, boosts your metabolism, assists in cell building, and is important to a healthy immune system. It also helps with weight loss, since the body requires a substantial amount of energy to break down protein.

You'll find protein in meat, fish, lentils, beans, egg, and dairy products like cottage cheese, cheese, and fat-free Greek yogurt.

Protein powder is a concentrated form of protein, and it absolutely has a place in your diet if you're strength training. Remember to buy the cleanest protein powder possible that is without any additives or unnecessary carbohydrates. Carbohydrates found in protein powders are typically fructose or glucose (table sugar). If you're eating a vegetarian diet, keep in mind that only 80 percent of vegetable protein is absorbed by the body, which is why I recommend that vegetarians take a protein supplement such as hemp powder or pea protein powder.

Obviously, there are different protein requirements among those who train and those who don't. If you're strength training, you'll need 0.06–0.07 oz (1.8–2 g) per 2.20 lbs (1 kg = 1000 g) of body weight daily. Remember that each meal should contain at least 0.70 oz (20 g) protein. The body can't store protein, so it's important to feed it protein at even intervals over time to optimize muscle growth. Protein provides 4 kilocalories per 0.03 oz (4 kcal/g).

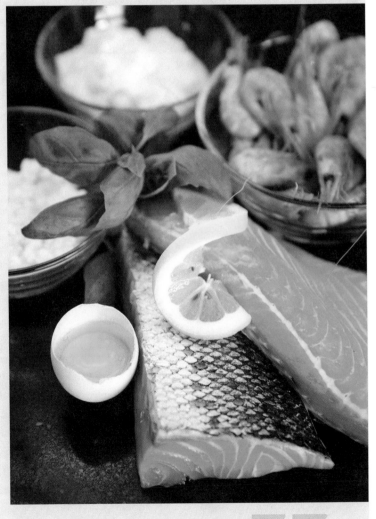

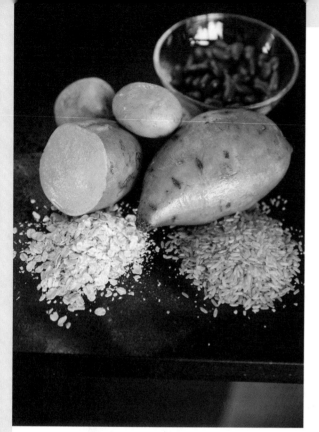

CARBOHYDRATES

Few nutrients cause as big a dilemma as to carb or not to carb. However, remember that if you're strength training you'll require more carbohydrates than if you're sedentary. And if you are serious about your training, you'll need carbohydrates because they provide you with the necessary energy for your workouts. Most carbohydrates are broken down by the body into glucose, a sugar used as fuel by the cells. Glucose is stored in the liver and in the muscles in the form of glycogen, which is used as backup energy for muscles and the brain.

Carbohydrates can be separated into fast- and slow-acting types, depending on how quickly they're broken down during digestion. Fast carbohydrates can cause sharp fluctuations in blood glucose levels, while slow-acting carbohydrates keeps blood glucose on an even keel and are therefore understood to be healthier for you. Take a look at the list from my pantry on page 37, which contains good quality, slow-acting carbohydrates.

One general guideline: Avoid sugar in all its guises, as it is not healthy.

Healthy nutritional fiber can be found in whole grains, root vegetables, legumes, vegetables, fruit, and berries. Fiber mostly passes through the body without being absorbed. Its primary purpose is to collect fluid and increase the volume in the intestine to prevent constipation. Fiber imparts feelings of fullness, and certain fibers positively affect insulin, cholesterol, and glucose levels in the blood. Try consuming 1–1¼ oz (25–35 g) of nutritional fiber a day, preferably from whole grain products, to make sure to reap those many benefits.

Some people are better able to deal with carbohydrates than others. Some can eat them and feel good and energetic while others feel their sweet tooth rearing its head; yet others become sluggish and sleepy. Find out what suits you, and adjust your diet accordingly.

Whatever goal we reach for, whether it is to have bigger muscles, less fat, or better aerobic capacity, we still need to replenish our fuel reserves with carbohydrates on a daily basis in order to feel well and to train at full capacity. Carbohydrates are our primary source of energy because all of our body's cells can use this particular fuel. If we don't consume enough carbohydrates, our fat deposits will start coming into play to provide, among other things, fuel for our brains. When the body gets too low on food-derived carbohydrates and glycogen deposits are depleted, the body starts to believe that it is starving. As a result, our fat-burning capacity will decrease while the breakdown of protein ramps up in the muscles. In other words, our hard-earned muscles are being consumed. For optimal fat burning, you'll need to eat an adequate daily amount of carbohydrates, at least 0.05–0.07 oz per 2.20 lbs (1.5–2 g per 1 kg) of body weight.

Carbohydrates provide 4 kilocalories per 0.03 oz (4 kcal/g).

FAT

Fat, much like carbohydrates, has recently come under the spotlight and its role debated. Our preoccupation is on the health effects of saturated versus unsaturated fats. I am not going to cover any specific diets in any great detail, since my interest lies more in how fat affects muscle growth and end goals.

Don't avoid fats because you think they are bad for you; however, the fats you do eat should be high in nutritional value. They will help you burn energy and absorb vitamins A, D, E, and K; they will also affect testosterone secretion, which is important for muscle development.

There are different types of fat: saturated, monounsaturated, and polyunsaturated. You'll find saturated fat in butter, cream, fatty meats, and cheeses. Monounsaturated fat is present in olive oil, canola oil, nuts, and avocados. Polyunsaturated fats feature in fatty fish such as salmon, mackerel, and smoked herring, as well as in seeds and flax oil. Polyunsaturated fats contain plenty of essential omega-3 and omega-6 fatty amino acids, which you'll ingest through eating food.

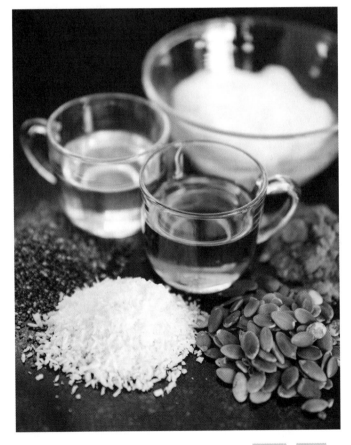

Trans-fatty acids (trans fats) are fats you should avoid because they raise levels of LDL cholesterol—the bad kind—in the blood. Trans fats are a natural part of beef and mutton, but you can also find them in some cookies and biscuits with long shelf lives, as well as in microwave popcorn, down-market margarines, snacks, powdered sauces, and more. Avoid them! And use my list of good fats on page 37 as a guide.

As for how much fat one should consume, 0.04–0.05 oz per 2.20 lbs (1.3–1.5 g per 1 kg) body weight per day is appropriate.

Fat provides 9 kilocalories per 0.03 oz (9 kcal/g).

ALCOHOL

I'm sure you've wondered about the effects of alcohol on training. Is it true that fat burning stops the moment you begin drinking? Well, as long as alcohol is present in the body, the fat burning process is put on hold. A bigger concern is that drinking tends to lift inhibitions, which in turns makes it too easy to start snacking on junk food.

This doesn't mean you should become a teetotaler, however—an occasional alcoholic drink is unlikely to cancel everything out. A glass of red wine now and then won't sabotage your training, as long as you don't overdo things.

WATER

It's important to drink enough water while you're training; you'll need 1½ quarts (1½ liters = 1500 ml) per day. Your glycogen stores will enable you to do more and go longer if you stay properly hydrated. It's natural to sweat while exercising as it is the body's way of cooling down; at the same time, sweating drains the body of fluids. Therefore, take care to drink more while training, preferably up to a quart (liter).

If you get hungry even though it hasn't been long since your last meal, it might be because you're thirsty. Drink a glass of water and see if you feel better.

Water also helps the body process the fiber in your food, since the fiber needs water to do its job.

If you feel that it's a chore to drink all that extra water, try sparkling water, or add in a twist of lemon or orange, some slices of cucumber, or strawberries.

MY PANTRY

Opt for organic produce as often as you can.

BEST SOURCES OF PROTEIN

- Feta cheese (10% fat)
- Pork tenderloin
- Turkey
- Cottage cheese
- Fat-free Greek yogurt
- Chicken
- Ground beef (5–10% fat)
- Salmon
- Mackerel
- Mozzarella (20% fat)
- Cheese (10% fat)
- Sirloin
- Shrimp
- Tofu
- Tuna
- Cod
- Game
- Eggs

BEST FATS

- 100% raw chocolate
- Avocado
- Chia seeds
- Fatty fish (salmon, mackerel, sardines, smoked Baltic herring)
- Fish oil
- Seeds (flax seeds, sunflower seeds, pumpkin seeds, etc.)
- Cocoa (preferably raw)
- Coconut oil
- Flax seed oil
- Nut butter (sugar and salt-free)
- Nuts (almonds, walnuts, etc.)
- Olives
- Olive oil
- Cold-pressed canola oil

- Grated coconut
- Butter (preferably unsalted)

BEST FRUITS/BERRIES

- Oranges
- Bananas
- Blueberries
- Grapefruit
- Raspberries
- Strawberries
- Kiwi fruit
- Plums
- Pears
- Apples

BEST SOURCES OF CARBOHYDRATES

- Buckwheat
- Beans/legumes
- Whole grain bread
- Rolled oats
- Potatoes
- Quinoa
- Root vegetables (parsnips, carrots, beets, rutabagas, etc.)
- Brown rice
- Sweet potatoes

BEST VEGETABLES

- Eggplant
- Avocadoes
- Cabbage (cauliflower, broccoli, kale, dinosaur/lacinato kale, white cabbage)
- Bell peppers
- Lettuce/mixed greens
- Asparagus

- Spinach
- Mushrooms
- Tomatoes
- Zucchini

BEST SEASONINGS

- Balsamic vinegar
- Lemon and lime juices
- Curry, red and green
- Cinnamon
- Cardamom
- Coconut milk
- Crushed tomatoes, without added sugar
- Marinated garlic cloves
- Gingerbread spices
- Pesto
- Salsa (without added sugar)
- Sambal oelek
- Mustard (without added sugar)
- Soy (low-sodium version)
- Mushrooms
- Tabasco hot sauce
- Garlic
- Apple sauce (without added sugar)

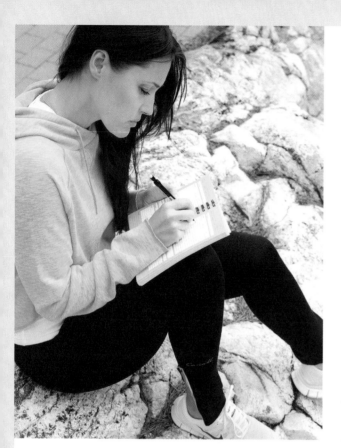

HOW DO YOU EAT WHILE TRAINING?

To optimize the benefits of your workouts, there are a few guidelines you should follow with regards to eating while you're training.

In brief: Opt for slow-acting carbohydrates (check the list of best carbohydrates from my pantry on page 37) and protein before the workout, and go for fast-acting carbohydrates and protein after exercise. This also applies if you train later in the day.

Before and right after a workout, avoid eating fat. Fat slows down your digestion, which is exactly the opposite of what you want to have happen after a workout because your body needs energy—and fast!

If you strength train first thing in the morning, never do so on an empty stomach; you need amino acids to prevent muscle breakdown. A protein drink, taken about 15 minutes before your workout, is perfect. Eat your normal breakfast after the workout, within 30 minutes.

If a power walk is your cardio routine, eat no food prior to your workout if it's in the morning, or go for your walk one hour after eating. As I've mentioned before, this is not that important if you go for the low intensity cardio. You don't need a recovery meal afterward; just eat normally as planned.

HOW TO EAT BEFORE A WORKOUT

Select slow-acting carbohydrates and protein, such as fruit and whole grain bread with cottage cheese. Give yourself enough time to eat before your workout—at least half an hour—so you have enough time to absorb the food. Make sure you're not hungry right before or during your exercise session.

Avoid sports drinks and any pure carbohydrates right before and during your workout.

HOW TO EAT AFTER A WORKOUT

You can go for fast-acting carbohydrates and easily digested protein. Good examples are a protein drink and a banana with an unsalted rice cake, or a ham sandwich and a smoothie made with natural yogurt and a banana.

The rule of thumb is to take in about 30 g (1 oz) carbohydrates and 20 g (⅔ oz) protein. Studies show that muscles grow and recover quicker when protein and carbohydrates are consumed together.

How soon prior to working should one eat? It varies from person to person, but try to keep your meal within 30 minutes to 1 hour of your training session. You'll need energy to perform! And if you're training you will also need food during your recovery period. Avoid fasting; that's not a good condition for building muscles or for recovery.

THE IMPORTANCE OF KEEPING A FOOD JOURNAL

A food journal can reveal far more than you may believe. I have read many food journals over the years, and I've realized that by analyzing their contents you can detect if one is consuming too little or too much of a particular nutrient. You can also observe how the rest of the day is affected if one skips breakfast; if a pattern of sweet tooth cravings emerges; how mood affects eating habits, and so on and so forth.

I hope you realize how important it is to keep a close eye on your eating habits. It's not just about writing down what you eat. If you analyze your notes, you'll learn more about how you feel and live, and you'll also figure out ways to avoid certain traps and improve your quality of life.

Check page 143 for an example of a food journal.

TRY WEIGHING YOUR FOOD

The advantage of weighing your food is that you can easily see how much of it you need to reach your goals. Many have trouble with portion sizes and have no idea what a proper portion looks like, so put some food on scales to get a better picture. I'm not suggesting that you continue to weigh your food forever—it's neither practical nor necessary—but you might want to keep it up for a few months so you develop good habits and discover what your meals should look like. If you want to try guessing how much your food weighs, test yourself by weighing an object like your mobile phone. First, guess its weight and then put it on the scales. How did you do? Now you'll know if your guesstimate is close enough.

WHAT HAPPENS IF YOU CRAVE SWEETS?

Craving sweets might indicate that your blood sugar level is too low, i.e., you're hungry or you haven't eaten enough. You can control these cravings more effectively if you always feel satiated, so check your calorie intake and follow the nutritional program meticulously. Be rigorous about eating some protein at every meal.

"What? I can't have even one dessert this entire time?"

Don't worry! Whatever you do, don't fret. I am against food rules that are too strict, because the more extreme you are, the greater you risk falling off the wagon. But you should be selective. If you're invited out for a meal on Saturday, go ahead and indulge, but then stay away from sweet treats on Sunday. You'll need to make a choice. My advice is to follow the 90/10 rule—if you eat healthy 90 percent of the time, you can indulge yourself during the remaining 10 percent, as long as it happens over one day and not several days. If you eat 42 times per week (6 times a day, both meals and snacks), you have the opportunity to enjoy something extra. Try this for one or two such meals per week. A good tip is to save your treat for nighttime—that way you're not tempted to run back to the refrigerator repeatedly. Many of us have trouble controlling our food intake once we give ourselves a little freedom. Be smart—become aware of your weaknesses, and avoid them!

Don't be tempted to quell your craving for sweets by eating something sweet, but if you cannot resist, start by drinking a large glass of water. If that doesn't do the trick, drink a cup of sweet-tasting (but unsweetened) herbal tea, eat a piece of fruit or a piece of dark chocolate. Remember—don't be too hard on yourself, and don't forget the 90/10 rule I mentioned earlier.

HOW TO EAT WELL WHEN EATING OUT

Do we have to give up altogether when we're on the road? Of course not. With a bit of planning, you'll always be prepared. The trick is to get a cooler bag, the perfect place to store your own food. You can find affordable ones at just about any store.

My best tips for eating out:

Drink 3 to 4 glasses of water before leaving the house; the fluid will fill you up.

- Eat a meal rich in protein with vegetables before going out. Protein will keep you satiated for a long time, and cravings for sweets are dampened when you feel full.
- Control your portions—stay within the size of your palm. Take just one bite of everything.

- Eat protein and vegetables first, and once you start feeling full you can then eat carbohydrates.
- Choose your treats carefully. Will it be dessert or alcohol? Remember that the more alcohol you consume, the more likely you'll eat more.
- No doggie bags! Share dessert with your partner or a friend. You can also order half a portion if you don't have anyone to share with.
- Work out on that day.

Don't forget that enjoying one's self and having fun doesn't always need to revolve around food.

HOW MANY CALORIES SHOULD YOU EAT?

I'm a firm believer in being aware of the number of calories you have to consume. It's important to differentiate between where calories come from and if those calories are beneficial to your health, your metabolism, and your goals. What will give you better results: a bowl full of potato chips or a snack packed with wholesome ingredients with the same amount of calories? Which is better for your health? To help you find out how many calories you need, calculate your BMR (basal metabolic rate; read more about it on page 20). Your calorie requirements will vary from step to step depending on where you are in the program, since muscle building, fine-tuning, and fat burning call for different amounts of calories. Below, you will find an approximate calculation of your basal calorie requirement, i.e., how much energy you need at rest. The formula applies to women:

(9.247 x weight in kilograms) + (3.098 x height in centimeters) - (4.330 x age) + 447.593 = BMR

1 inch = 2.54 cm
1 kilogram = 2.2 lbs

Now, multiply your BMR by the appropriate level of activity:

Sedentary or very little training	1.2
Light training (1–3 times/week)	1.375
Moderate training (3–5 times/week)	1.55
Intense training (6–7 times/week)	1.725
High intensity training (2 times/day)	1.9

The number that comes up will be the calorie requirement for keeping your weight stable. Keep in mind that if your weight (or age) changes, you'll have to recalculate your BMR.

NUTRIENT DISTRIBUTION

The best and smartest way to extract the most nutrients from food is to allot various nutrients over mealtimes. Here is a good starting point, with an example on how to do the calculation. Check my recipes (starting on page 49) to see what a good distribution of proteins, carbohydrates, and fat looks like.

As mentioned before, protein requirements for people who work out are approximately 0.07 oz (2 g) per 2.20 lbs of body weight. So if you weigh 154.5 lbs (70 kg), you'll need approximately 5 oz (140 g) protein a day.

An adequate level of fat is 0.03–0.04 oz (1–1.3 g) per 2.20 lbs of body weight. If you get enough essential fatty acids, which you will almost always do if you follow my nutritional advice, your fat intake need not be much higher. Fat makes food taste better because many flavors are fat soluble, and you also need to absorb fat-soluble vitamins.

We have now calculated how much protein and fat you need, so it is now quite simple to add in the carbohydrates to reach your total calorie requirement (see the example below). Don't forget that carbohydrate requirements for someone who works out are higher than for someone who doesn't exercise, so don't lower the amount of carbs too much. If you include carbohydrates in your meal plan, you'll have the stamina for more intense workouts, and you will recover from them more efficiently.

Remember that 0.03 oz (1 g) protein and 0.03 oz (1 g) carbohydrate are 4 kilocalories (kcal), while 0.03 oz (1 g) fat is 9 kilocalories (kcal).

Example:
- A person who weighs 154.5 lbs (70 kg) needs 1,830 kilocalories (kcal).
- Protein intake should be approximately 5 oz (140 g) per day = 560 kilocalories (kcal).
- Fat intake should be between 2.5 oz (70 g) and 3.2 oz (90 g); let's say 2.8 oz (80 g) for simplicity's sake = 720 kilocalories (kcal).
- Now fill up on carbohydrates [1830—(560 + 720)], which in this case comes to = 550 kilocalories (kcal) or 4.85 oz (137.5 g).

Now it will be easy to create your meal plan. Allot your required amounts of protein, fat, and carbohydrate over the day's meals. If you're going to divvy up 5 oz (140 g) of protein over 5 meals, you'll end up with 1 oz (28 g) per meal. You can get 1 oz (28 g) of protein in a 4.25 oz (120 g) chicken breast, for instance, or in a 5.8 oz (164 g) fillet of cod.

It's not the end of the world if you don't like an even distribution of nutrients between your daily meals or if eat more at lunch or dinner and less at breakfast, as long as the total amount is fairly close. Try to space your daily food intake as evenly as you can throughout the day to avoid energy flags.

You've now calculated your nutritional needs. Keep in mind that this figure is approximate, since your activity levels will vary from day to day. You might not be feeling well, you might have to travel, or perhaps you can't work out as you'd planned for some other reason.

Evaluate your results after a few weeks. If you have followed the plan and have nothing to show for it, check that you are following the training program properly and maybe adjust your calorie intake depending on which step you are at. If you want to lose fat, eat fewer calories. If you want to increase your muscle mass instead but see no results even after training correctly, eat more calories.

NUTRITION FOR STEP 1: **BUILDING**

Return to page 41 where you calculated your daily calorie needs, and add 500 kilocalories to the sum you ended up with. This is to ensure muscle growth at this step. If you find it difficult to eat that much, tack on the 500 calories progressively at your own speed; don't eat it all in one go.

A few tips

- Avoid all obvious sources of sugar. You'll be well on your way if you do this.
- Get rid of all the junk food from your home. If it's at home, you will eat it sooner or later. You should be aware of your weaknesses and pitfalls, so clean out all the junk from your pantry and refrigerator. Do not take this opportunity to eat the candy you find because it is going in the trash anyway; throw it away immediately—right now!
- Plan ahead. To eat the right way, you can start by changing the type of foods you buy. It's easy to start off being too strict, only to get burnt out. Focus on one thing at a time. For example, shop for your weekly meals on Saturdays, prepare your to-go meals, and plan your workout schedule on Sundays. Not everything has to be locked up in one day.
- Avoid going all out. Extreme diets aren't sustainable—and you are looking to change the way you live, aren't you? Concentrate on good food that will help you build muscles and keep you satiated. You'll need to feel good, have the energy for your workouts, and keep yourself going throughout the day.

Your task now is to stock your home with food from the list of suggested ingredients on page 37. You'll ace it! Honestly, I'm convinced that your entire family will benefit from eating the same food as you.

NUTRITION FOR STEP 2: **FINE-TUNING**

As you're still building muscles at this stage, you can continue with the same calorie intake as in Step 1, i.e., your daily calorie allowance + 500 kilocalories (kcal). Remember to adjust it if you see any change in body weight.

Time to evaluate Step 1
- How are you doing? Have you seen any improvement? Or rather, do you feel it?
- Do you feel energetic during the workouts and for the rest of the day?
- Are you staying on track with the food I recommended, at least 90 percent of the time?
- Are you in control over the weekend, or do you tend to fall off the wagon, nutritionally speaking?

Bear in mind that every small piece of bread and each square of chocolate counts, as does the extra spoonful of nut butter. These can make the number of calories mount up over a single week.

If you feel that you haven't seen any progress, look into this
- If you ate something not on the recommended list, was it a craving or were you just unprepared and hungry?
- How about your protein intake? Are you consuming your allotted amount at each meal? If not, go back and reread the section on protein so you don't forget.
- How much water do you drink?
- How is your stomach feeling? Are you feeling any stress?
- Do you get enough sleep?

Mull over these questions, and if you don't notice any changes, reflect on your food choices. You might need to make some tweaks somewhere.

NUTRITION FOR STEP 3: **BURNING**

We will now return to page 41 to calculate your caloric needs, but we're not going to add any extra calories. Instead we're going to remove some and keep up a slight caloric deficit, the purpose being to reduce your adipose fat without losing too much muscle mass in the process.

Take your calculated calorie requirement (remember to adjust it for any possible weight changes) and reduce that amount by 350 to 500 kilocalories (kcal). Your body needs a minimum of 1,550 kilocalories (kcal) per day for essential vitamins, minerals, fatty acids, and amino acids, but you should not refer to this number when you are strength training.

NUTRITION—CONCLUSION

Remember that the ultimate goal of making good food choices is to feel better, to do more in your workouts, and to have energy for everyday living. You are not going to be counting calories forever, but you are laying the groundwork for food habits that will sustain you long after you've finished this book.

• Make sure to eat protein at each meal.
• Eat regularly.
• Eat carbohydrates before or after a workout—they'll help you recover and give you energy.
• Don't forget to include wholesome fats and vegetables at most meals.
• Keep a food journal.

For more help along the way, refer to the recipes starting on page 49 for all your daily meals.

MY FAVORITE RECIPES

It's very important for me that food preparation doesn't take too long. Like you, my days are filled with too many things to do. To make things easier for myself, I make sure my refrigerator and pantry are always stocked with healthy staples, which you can find in my top pantry lists (page 37). I can pick and mix from among those groups as I please, being certain that I will always enjoy good, wholesome food. You simply can't go wrong if you follow my ingredients list.

I'm often asked if our children eat like we do. The answer is yes—they partake in about 80 percent of the same food we eat. Off my ingredients list, they might not like beans, lentils, and sweet potato, but they gobble up everything else with gusto. We were always careful to not feed our kids from a separate menu. They were expected to taste every dish first and to not reject food outright. However, we have never forced them to eat anything they do not like.

A good thing would be to find some favorite food items that can be made into quick, tasty meals, such as fat-free Greek yogurt. Fat-free Greek yogurt is one of the best heath foods around because it's packed with protein, it's very filling, and it contains few calories. You can also use it in a variety of ways: combine it with berries and fruit, use it as dip or a base for a cold sauce, or add it to smoothies. Other on-the-go meals include mackerel in tomato sauce, hardboiled eggs, different types of omelets, or cold crêpes that you can stuff with cottage cheese, grated apple, honey, and cinnamon.

Don't forget to eat about six meals a day:

Breakfast
Snack 1
Lunch
Snack 2
Dinner
Snack 3

On page 49, you'll find my favorite recipes for breakfast, lunch, snacks, and dinner. Note: these are individual recipes that are examples of good food, but they do not comprise a full meal plan. Each recipe includes the calorie count and the nutritional breakdown of protein, carbohydrates, and fats. Each recipe serves one.

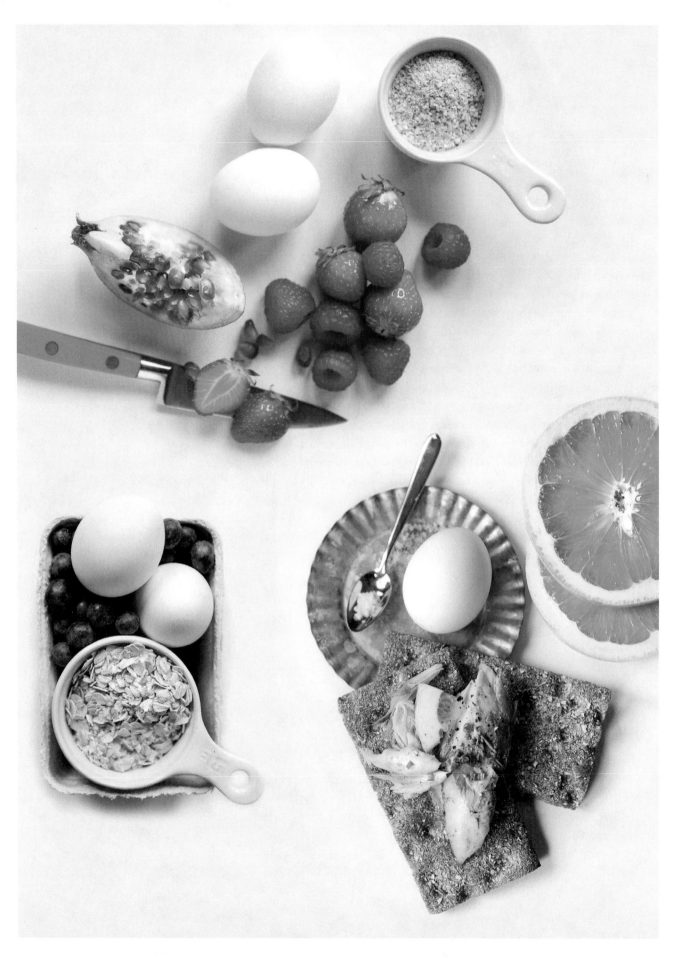

OATMEAL WITH BLUEBERRIES AND CINNAMON

This is my standard breakfast. Not only does it make me feel full the entire morning, it's also cheap to make!

352 kcal—C 29.7 g—P 20.2 g—F 15.4 g

¾ cup water
½ cup rolled oats
½ cup frozen blueberries
Ground cinnamon
2 large eggs, hard-boiled

Bring the water and oats to a boil, and then let simmer for a few minutes.

Place the blueberries at the bottom of a soup bowl, spoon the oatmeal on top, and season with cinnamon. Serve with two boiled eggs.

OAT CRÊPES

Try my oat crêpes if you need a change from oatmeal. They're easy to cook and also make a handy portable snack.

462 kcal—C 37.4 g—P 27.9 g—F 20.2 g

4 tbsp oat bran
4 tbsp fat-free Greek yogurt
2 large eggs
1 tsp coconut oil
½ cup berries
1 apple

Mix oat bran, yogurt, and eggs to make a batter. Cook the crêpes in coconut oil.

Enjoy the crêpes with berries and an apple on the side.

TIP! You can also serve the crêpes with 1 oz (30 g) smoked salmon and 2 tbsp of sauce made from yogurt and roe. Top with fresh dill.

POWER BREAKFAST with mackerel, egg, and grapefruit

Breakfast doesn't always have to be oatmeal. Why not try something totally different, for high energy and nourishment!

466 kcal—C 41.3 g—P 23 g—F 21.4 g

1 large hard-boiled egg
2 slices of hard rye (e.g., Wasa)
1¾ oz (50 g) smoked mackerel
1 grapefruit

Slice the egg with an egg slicer and place it on one of the slices of crisp bread. Put strips of mackerel on the other slice.

Serve the open-faced sandwiches with grapefruit.

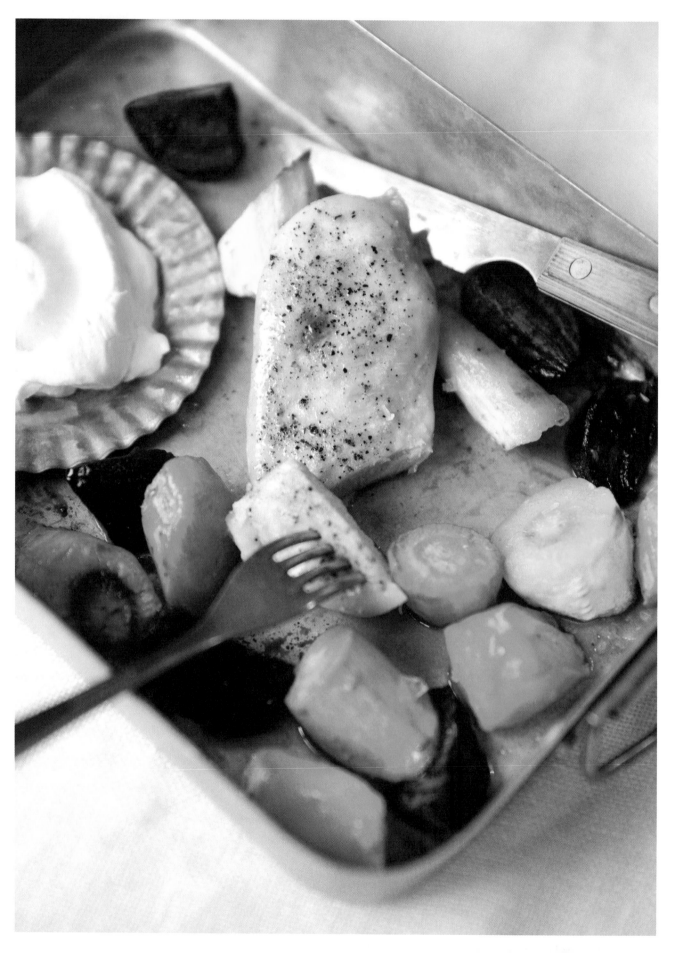

CHICKEN with roasted root vegetables and goat cheese crème

Root vegetables are a great source of carbohydrates. If you want to avoid gluten, give this dish a try!

336 kcal—C 21.3 g—P 30.3 g—F 12.7 g

1 carrot
1 beet
1 parsnip
1 tsp olive oil
Salt and freshly ground black pepper
3½ oz (100 g) chicken breast
1 oz goat cheese
1 tbsp low-fat milk

Preheat the oven to 390°F (200°C).

Peel and cut the root vegetables in large chunks. Transfer them to an ovenproof dish or a rimmed baking sheet, and toss the vegetables in olive oil, salt, and pepper.

Set the dish in the oven for 15 minutes, and then add in the chicken breast. Cook for another 15 to 20 minutes.

Mash the goat cheese with the milk.

Transfer the root vegetables and chicken to a plate. Add dollops of goat cheese crème and serve.

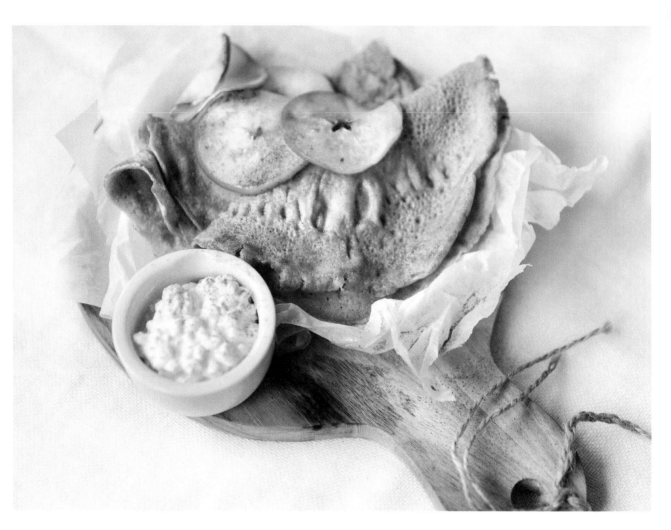

BUCKWHEAT CRÊPES with cottage cheese and cooked apple

These crêpes are just as good for breakfast, lunch, or dinner. If you're lucky, the kids will love them, too!

471 kcal—C 21.4 g—P 16.3 g—F 58.2 g

¾ cup almond milk, unsweetened
½ cup buckwheat flour
1 pinch salt
2 large eggs
1 tsp (5 g) coconut oil
½ apple
1 pinch ground cinnamon
2 tbsp cottage cheese (4% fat)

Mix half the almond milk with the buckwheat flour and salt, and whisk until you have a smooth batter. Whisk in the eggs and the remaining almond milk. Whisk until the batter is smooth. Let the batter rest for 5 minutes.

Fry the crêpes in a skillet with melted coconut oil.

Slice the apple and add it to the frying pan. Season with cinnamon and cook the apple slices until they've softened a little.

Serve the crêpes with cottage cheese, and top with the apple slices.

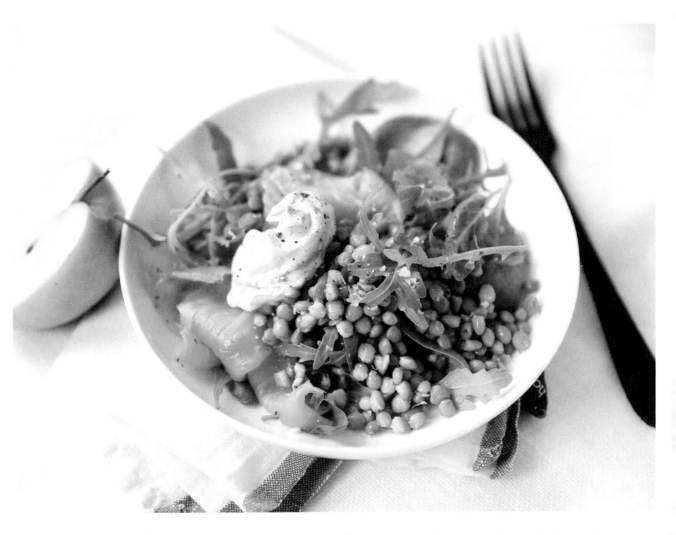

GRAVAD (RAW MARINATED) SALMON with red lentils

Salmon is one of my favorite sources of protein and nutrition, all in one ingredient. I could eat salmon every day without getting bored. This is a simple dish that can be made as easily at home or at work.

465 kcal—C 21.4 g—P 22.2 g—F 31.6 g

¼ cup Greek yogurt
1 tsp sambal oelek
½ cup red lentils, cooked
1¾ oz (50 g) marinated salmon
½ oz (10 g) spinach
Arugula
½ apple

Mix yogurt and sambal oelek.
Transfer the lentils, salmon and the yogurt mix to a plate.
Serve with spinach and arugula, with apple on the side.

LUNCH OMELET

In this dish I'm using mostly egg whites to boost the protein content. The fats come from avocado, olive oil, and feta cheese instead of from egg yolks; that way I can keep the calories under control. However, if you prefer making the omelet with whole eggs, use 3 large eggs and leave out the avocado.

401 kcal—C 22 g—P 21.4 g—F 23.4 g

1 large egg
4 large egg whites
1 tsp olive oil, for frying
2 oz (55 g) avocado, chopped
1¾ oz (50 g) cherry tomatoes, halved, approx. 5
4 tsp (20 g) feta cheese (10% fat), cubed
Fresh basil
2 kiwis

Mix the whole egg with the whites, and pour into a warm skillet coated with olive oil. Let the egg mix settle.

Add the avocado, tomatoes, and feta cheese on top, and top with basil leaves.

Serve with two kiwis.

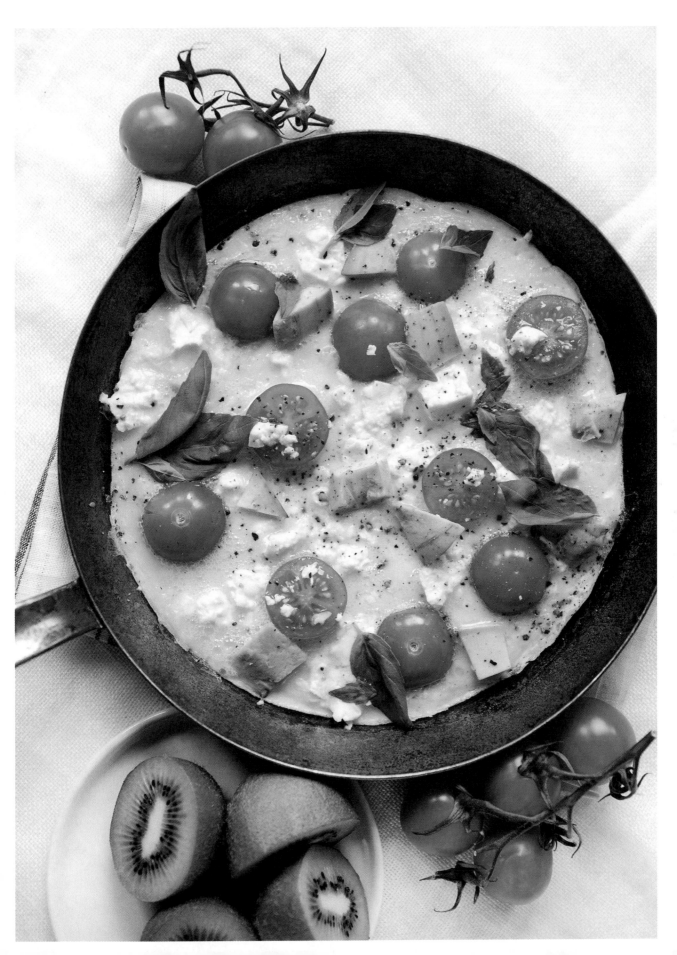

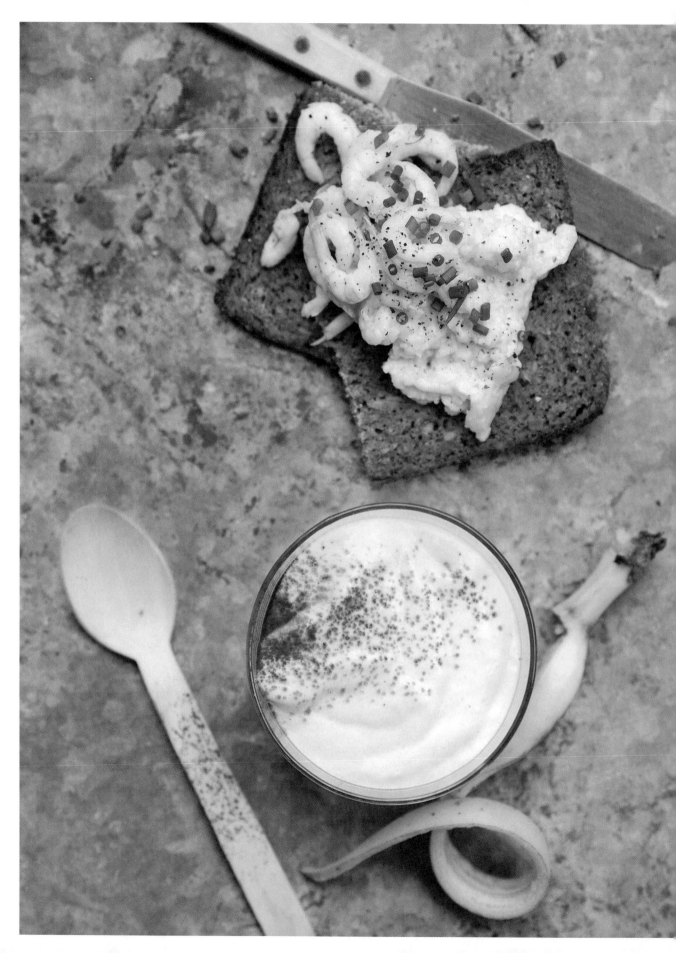

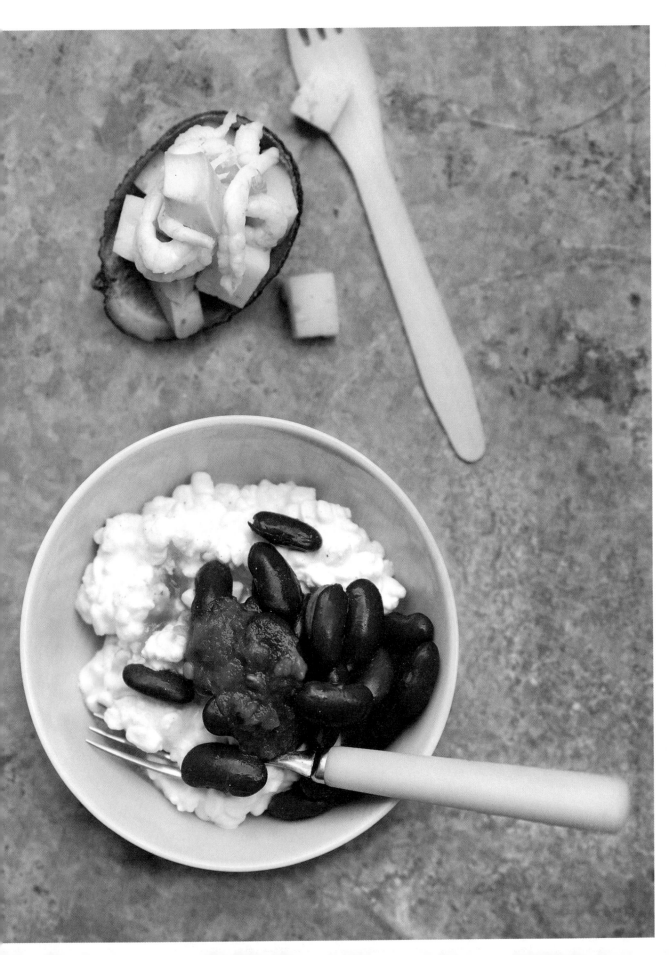

SNACKS

WHOLE GRAIN RYE BREAD with scrambled egg and shrimp

Bread is not a bad choice when you're looking to become fit, and here is a recipe that has it all. As usual, it's also a breeze to make.

339 kcal—C 23.6 g—P 22.47 g—F 15.34 g

1 tsp olive oil
1 large egg
1 slice of whole grain rye bread
(e.g., bread with 70% whole
grain rye)
1⅓ oz (40 g) shrimp, peeled

Heat the olive oil in a skillet, and scramble the egg.
Top the slice of bread with the scramble eggs and the shrimp.

YOGURT with banana ice cream and cinnamon

I always freeze overripe bananas. They're perfect for making tasty ice cream that even the kids will love. This snack illustrates what a post-workout meal might look like.

251 kcal—C 30.1 g—P 25.1 g—F 3.4 g

1 banana, frozen
¾ cup Greek yogurt
1 tsp ground cinnamon, and
maybe some cocoa

Blend the banana in a mixer until it takes on the texture of ice cream. Place the yogurt in a deep plate, top with the banana ice cream, and season with cinnamon and cocoa.

TIP! Try topping the ice cream with 1 tsp of peanut butter.

SHRIMP, CHEESE CUBES, AND AVOCADO

This is a simple snack that can be thrown together in 5 minutes. The healthy fat comes from avocado, and the protein from shrimp and cheese.

247 kcal—C 3.0 g—P 31.6 g—F 11.5 g

½ avocado
3½ oz (100 g) shrimp,
peeled
1 oz cheese (10% fat)

Remove the avocado flesh without breaking the skin, and chop.
   Mix shrimp, cheese, and avocado together, and fill the avocado's skin with the mix.

COTTAGE CHEESE with kidney beans and salsa

This is another favorite snack I've been enjoying from as far back as ten years ago, when my interest in strength training began.

256 kcal—C 11.9 g—P 28.6 g—F 9.5 g

¾ cup cottage cheese
¼ cup kidney beans, cooked
1–2 tbsp salsa, unsweetened,
from a jar

Place the cottage cheese on a plate and top with beans and salsa. Enjoy!

DINNER

SALMON BURGER with oven-baked sweet potato

Sweet potatoes have become one of my favorite foods, and so they turn up often in my meals. There isn't much difference between a sweet potato and a regular potato apart from sweet potato's nutritional value, which is slightly higher thanks to the orange color imparted by its high carotene content—the same element you find in carrots.

417 kcal—C 22 g—P 29 g—F 23.3 g

1 sweet potato
Salt
Freshly ground black pepper
Fresh thyme
4½ oz (125 g) salmon
1 standard-sized egg
¼ tsp saffron
1 tsp olive or coconut oil
⅓ oz (10 g) spinach

Preheat the oven to 400°F (200°C).

Cut the potato into fries, season them with salt and pepper, and transfer them to a baking sheet lined with parchment paper. Bake them in the oven for approximately 20 minutes or until the potatoes have turned brown. When the potatoes are ready, season them with thyme.

Cut the salmon into small chunks and mix with the egg. Season with saffron, salt, and pepper. Shape into burgers, and fry them in oil in a warm pan over medium heat.

Serve the salmon with the sweet potatoes, and garnish with spinach.

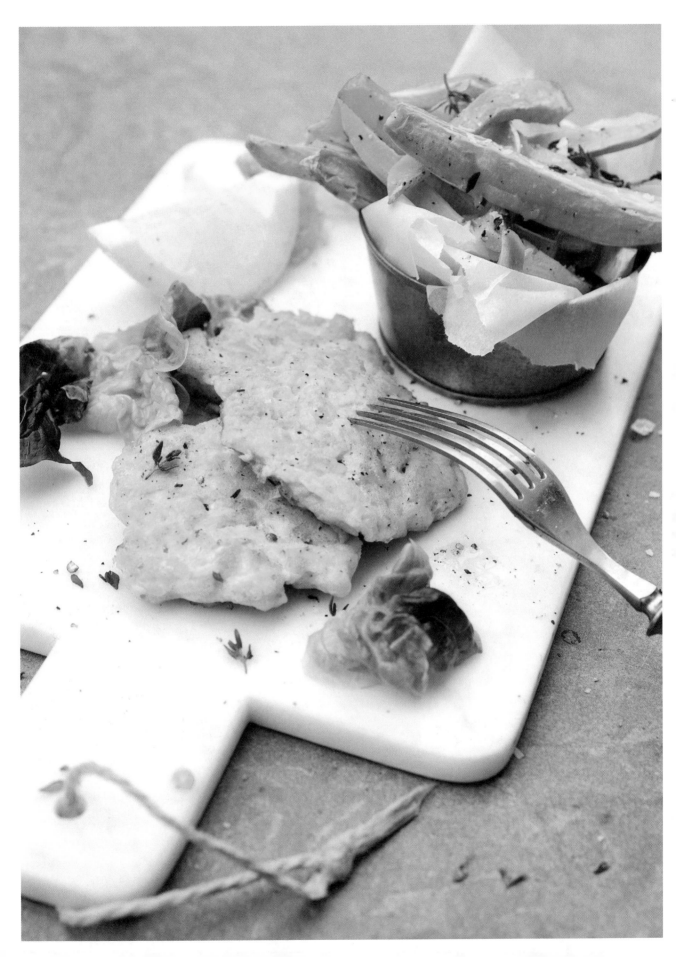

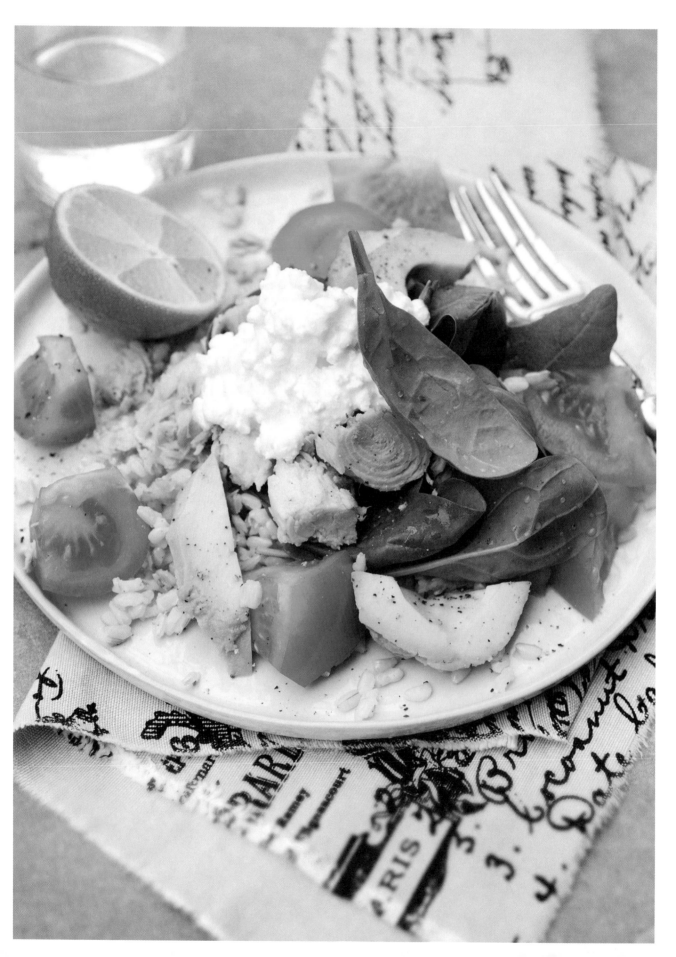

TUNA with brown rice and vegetables

Tuna doesn't have to be boring and eaten straight from the can. Try this recipe and, suddenly, eating tuna will become a whole new experience!

423 kcal—C 38.2 g—P 36.4 g—F 13 g

3½ oz (100 g) water-packed tuna
½ cup brown rice, cooked
¼ cup cottage cheese
½ avocado
⅓ oz (10 g) spinach
1 tomato, cut into wedges
1 tsp lime juice
A pinch of herb salt

Drain the tuna. Place the tuna, rice, cottage cheese, avocado, spinach, and tomato on a plate.

Squeeze some lime juice over the fish, and season the cottage cheese with the herb salt.

STUFFED CABBAGE, the lazy way

This is a favorite dish from my childhood; I still make it and it never gets old.

452 kcal—C 44 g—P 29.7 g—F 16.6 g

4¼ oz (120 g) ground beef (10–12% fat)
1 tsp cold-pressed canola oil
3½ oz (100 g) white cabbage, shredded
½ onion, chopped
Salt and freshly ground black pepper
½ cup brown rice, cooked

Sauté the beef in oil until the meat has browned slightly.

Add the cabbage and the onion to the pan with the beef. Combine and keep cooking, covered, for 5 to 7 minutes, stirring occasionally until the white cabbage has softened. Season it with salt and pepper.

Stir in the rice and serve.

TIP! As my husband does, serve the stuffed cabbage with a tablespoon of lingonberry or cranberry preserves.

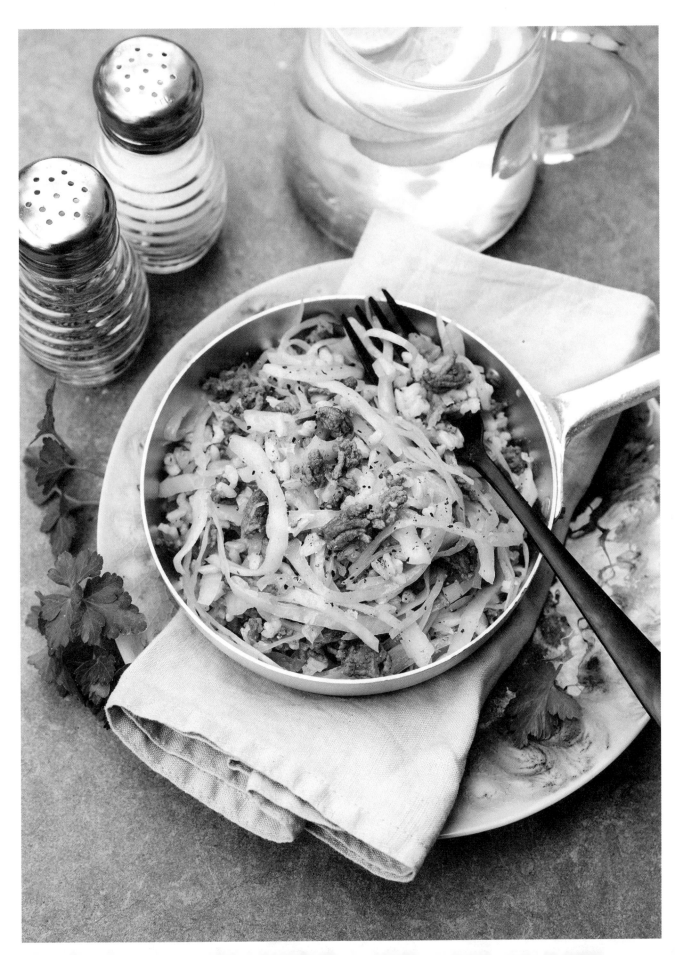

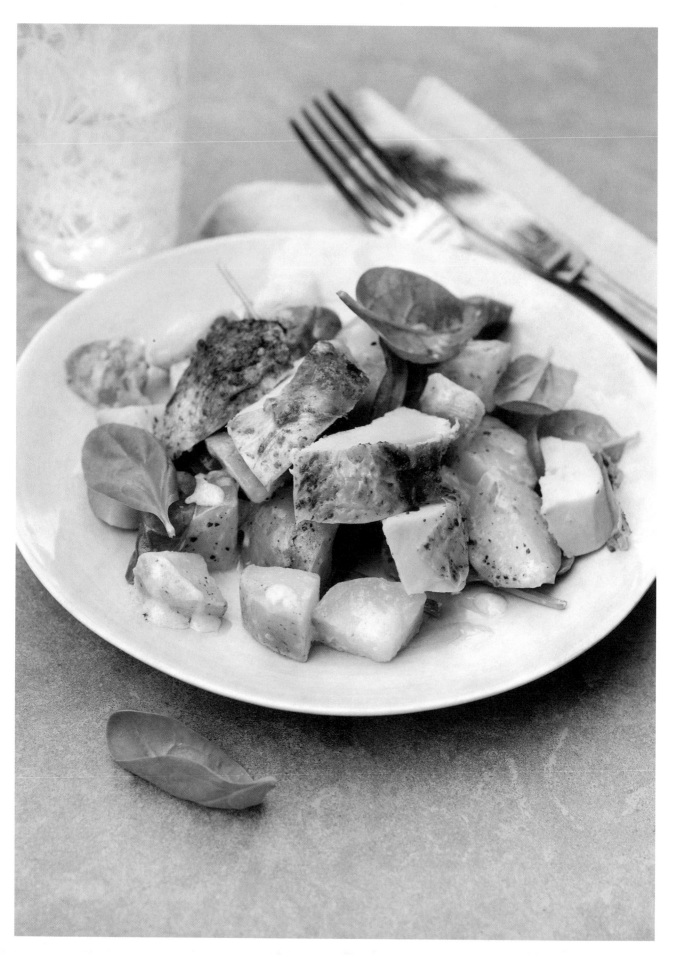

GRILLED CHICKEN with mustard potatoes

A flavorful dish that can be prepared in just a few minutes!

455 kcal—C 19.6 g—P 33.5 g—F 26.6 g

1 tbsp Dijon mustard
1 tsp olive oil
1 tbsp lemon juice
3 potatoes, cooked, cooled,
and unpeeled
⅓ oz (10 g) spinach
3½ oz (100 g) chicken,
grilled (with skin)

Make a dressing from the mustard, olive oil, and lemon juice.

Cut the potatoes into smaller chunks, and mix with the spinach and dressing.

Serve with the chicken.

BAKED SWEET POTATO with mix of chickpea and feta cheese

This is a perfect dish for vegetarians as feta cheese and chickpeas are both healthy sources of vegetarian protein.

475 kcal—C 59.7 g—P 17.9 g—F 15.7 g

1 8–10½ oz (250–300 g) sweet potato, raw, unpeeled
½ onion
1 garlic clove, crushed
1 tsp olive oil
⅓ cup chickpeas, cooked
⅓ oz (10 g) spinach
1 tbs lemon juice
Salt and freshly ground black pepper
1¾ oz (50 g) feta cheese (10% fat)

Preheat the oven to 475°F (250°C).

Bake the sweet potato until soft. Cut it in half lengthwise. You'll only need one half of the potato, so set aside the second half for lunch or for dinner the next day.

In a skillet over medium heat, sauté the onion and garlic in olive oil until softened. Add in the chickpeas and cook for a few more minutes.

Now stir in the spinach and add the lemon juice; season with salt and pepper.

Make a big hole in the sweet potato, fill it with the chickpea mixture, and top it with feta cheese.

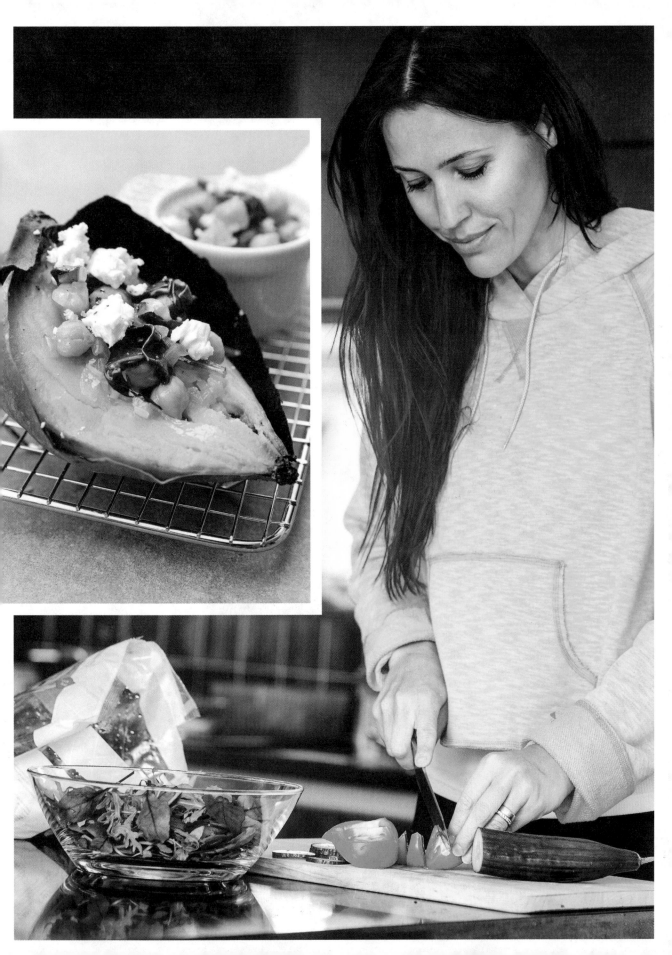

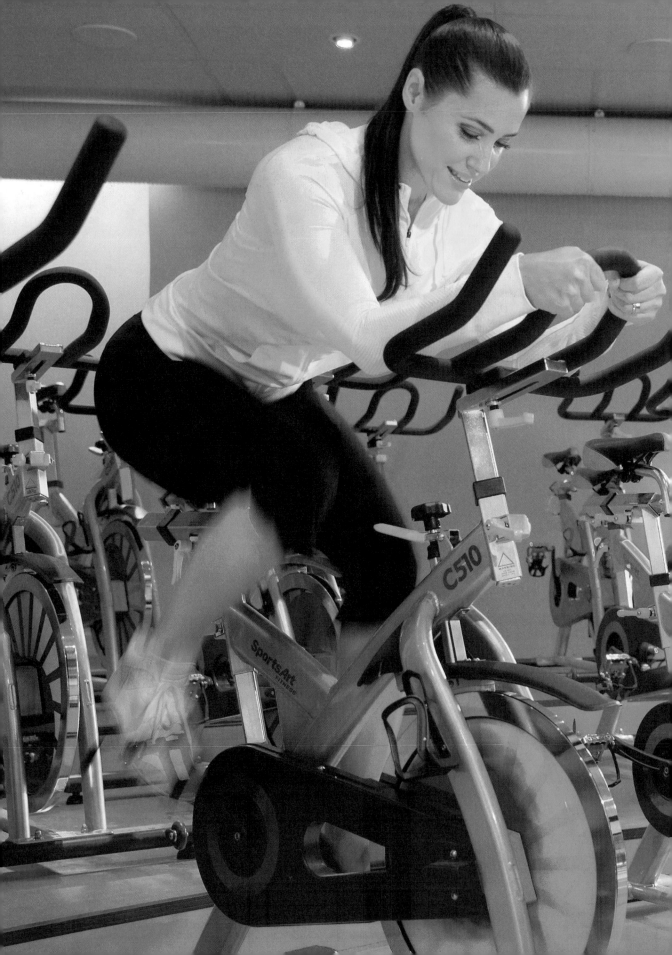

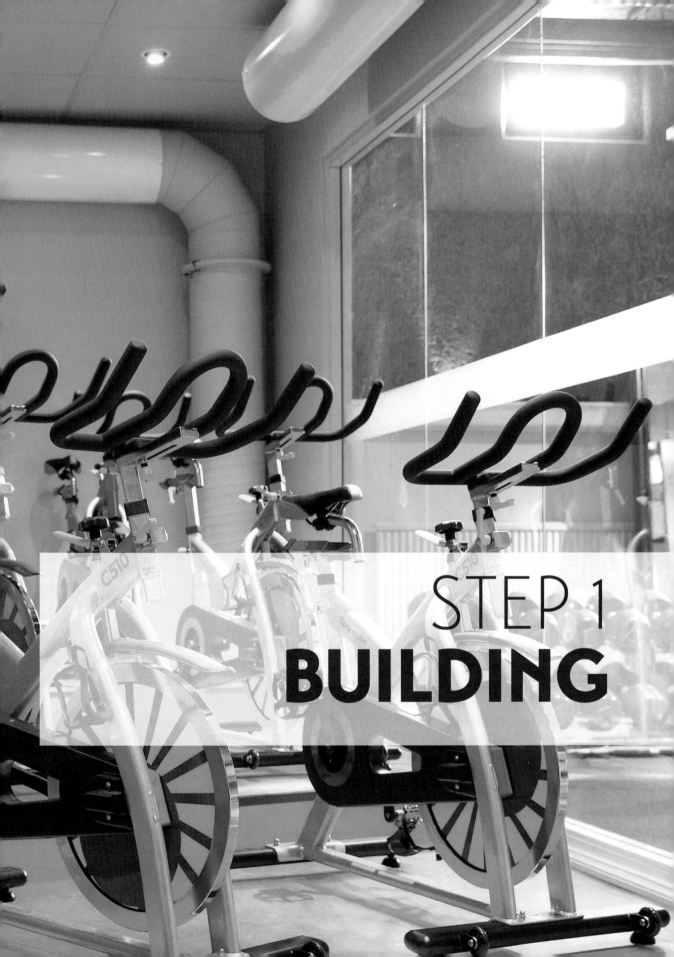

STEP 1
BUILDING

TIME TO DEVELOP NEW HABITS!

If you want a new body, identifythe steps you'll have to take to make it happen. Ask yourself: What habits do I need to develop in order for this to work? Be very specific. How should you train? At what time of the day should you exercise? Saying "I'm going to the gym," is too fuzzy; "I'll be at the gym on Wednesdays at 7:00 pm to do my strength training" is much more decisive. Eliminate any obstacles that could prevent you from reaching your goals. Remove commitments that could interfere with your workout schedule. Let family and friends know that this workout time is vital, and that you need to focus on your training.

Make sure you have a gym membership or all the equipment necessary for working out at home. It's fine to be eager, but it won't do you any good if you're left standing there, suddenly finding out you're missing elements key to achieving your goals.

Be patient. You'll need lots of perseverance. And even if you do notice positive results from the onset, they will eventually level out. And that's when you'll have to hang in there.

Around the sixth week of training, things are going to start feeling like a drag. Motivation will take a dive and you'll feel uninspired. At this point I say, "The honeymoon period is over." The novelty has worn off, and you realize you'll have to keep working out to keep seeing results. This is when the real challenge begins. And you aren't a failure simply because you miss a workout—you're human, life happens, and occasionally priorities get shuffled around.

If you find it difficult to get your motivation back, try a 30-day challenge. This period of time is long enough for you to establish a few good habits. And when you are successful 30 days in a row, that will surely be plenty enough to make you keep going on day 31, 32, and 45. You'll receive positive feedback from the progress you make, and that will keep happening as long as you keep up these new habits. You can't always muster the enthusiasm when thinking about working out for 365 days; it's much easier to break it up into shorter time frames lasting 7, 14, or 30 days at a time. Then it becomes difficult to stop. What, give up after 238 days? *No way!*

WHAT TO REMEMBER WHILE WORKING OUT

How much you're able to lift will depend to a certain extent on how you are feeling that particular day. If you haven't slept well the night before, you'll probably lift less weight; but if you're happy and feeling energetic, don't hesitate—go for it.

Don't use the same weight throughout your entire workout as this is neither effective nor smart. For instance, if you are performing back and chest exercises, you'll be able to hoist considerably heavier weights than when you are doing arm exercises. If you can lift equally heavy weights for a biceps curl as for a lying dumbbell press, then it's likely that your dumbbells are too light.

The last two to three repetitions of each set should be challenging to complete; nevertheless, don't forget to use proper form with each exercise so you don't end up injuring yourself. If your form suffers, lessen the weight at once; do not wait until the next workout. If you feel that you can do more reps than what the program tells you to, well, then your weights are too light. Do you feel you can handle heavier weights? Then increase the weight. Is your mind wandering—are you starting to plan dinner? Increase the weight.

Do you find it difficult to get in touch with your muscles? If so, it's time to check your form, and only increase the weight when everything feels right.

Proper form is critical. It's better to perform an exercise with weights that allow you finish all the reps than to use weights that lead you to lose proper form and risk injuring yourself. Avoid jerking movements, and strive to make them smooth and controlled. How you lift is as important as how much you lift. Count to yourself: up for 1 (lifting the weight), down for 2 to 3 (lowering the weight). Rest periods between sets should take about 1 minute when you work out with heavy weights. If you rest for less time, you probably won't be able to lift as much during your next set, but increase your rest a bit if you feel that your recovery time is too short between sets.

Try to control your breathing when you work out, and imagine that it's actually helping you lift the weight: exhale as you lift the weight, and inhale as you lower it.

It is imperative that you stand and sit correctly as you perform these exercises. Remember to keep your back in a neutral position (not slouched forward, not arched too far back). In a neutral position, your body works optimally without compressing the spine's vertebrae, you breathe more easily, your circulation increases, and your risk for injuries lessens. Use the same stance for the pelvis as if you were zipping up your pants—pull your navel inward toward the spine, and tilt your pelvis upward.

WORKOUT ROUTINE

Strength training consists of the basic exercises in step 1. It's important to start here because these moves will make you use your entire body. This will build the foundation you need to be able to progress on to the next steps. These compound movements engage several muscle groups and develop functional strength; you will hone your body's balance and teach your muscles to work together efficiently.

When lifting heavy weights, you need to use correct form. Compound movements require control; otherwise, you could become injured. It's important that you follow each exercise's directions to the letter and that you start off using lighter weights until you can perform the exercises correctly. For example, if you perform a dead lift, you need to pay attention to your core and back; and for this you will have to have worked on your core muscles. Once you've mastered the form, the weight you use should be heavy to the point where you can just manage the number of repetitions I have indicated for each exercise.

This program is designed to work both at home and in a gym, with the exception of the Pull-Down exercise (page 85) and Rowing Machine or Bent Over Row (page 84). Do the exercise if you have access to the machine; otherwise, give it a miss.

The exercises' descriptions begin on page 76; workout routines and weekly schedules can be found on page 132. The weekly schedule plans out your strength training and cardio work sessions, as well as rest days. And by rest day, I don't mean you should spend that time vegging out on the couch—why not try some yoga? It's perfect for keeping your body flexible and spry.

HOW LONG DOES THIS STEP LAST?

I recommend that this building period run for eight weeks. You might think it's going to be boring or unbalanced, but allow me to disagree: it will be neither of those things if you focus your energy on becoming better at lifting heavier weights, and your body will reward you by becoming stronger and stronger. Performing the same routine offers you the great advantage of not having to figure out what to do and how to do it every time, which makes for a more effective workout.

CARDIO FOR STEP 1

The objective of cardio training during this building phase is to keep up your level of general fitness and improve insulin sensitivity. Low intensity cardio is best, when building muscles is the main objective. Walk, bike, or swim at a moderate pace without getting too winded (read more about low intensity cardio on pages 26–27).

I prefer to keep cardio and strength training sessions apart. Doing cardio work on rest days is good because it turns into active recovery and allows you to burn a few calories.

WARM UP

I make a point of using dynamic warm-ups; this prepares muscles for
the work ahead.

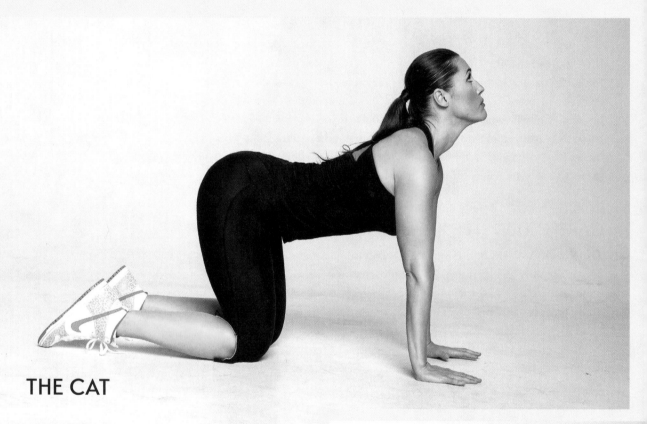

THE CAT

Position yourself on the floor on all fours; your
hands are under your shoulders.
Breathe in through your nose; keep your back
in the neutral position while pressing your chest
forward and looking up toward the ceiling. Breathe
out through your mouth, arch your back, and look
in toward your stomach.

- 1 x 15
- **Warms up:** The spine.

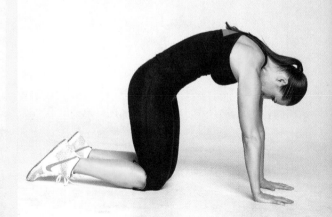

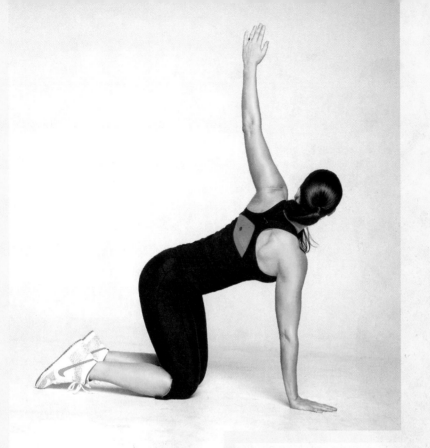

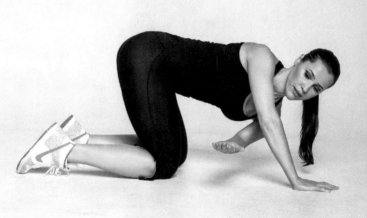

THREADING THE NEEDLE—OPEN ARM VARIATION

Stay on your hands and knees, hands aligned under your shoulders. Bring one arm out to your side, then up and back as far as you can reach. Look back at your hand, and then bring it back down and under your body, palm pointing up, bending slightly at the knees and jutting the buttocks backward.

• 1 x 15 on each side
• **Warms up:** Upper back, spine, and shoulders.

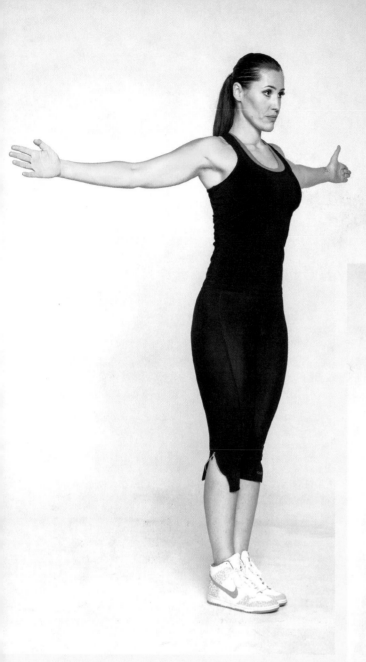
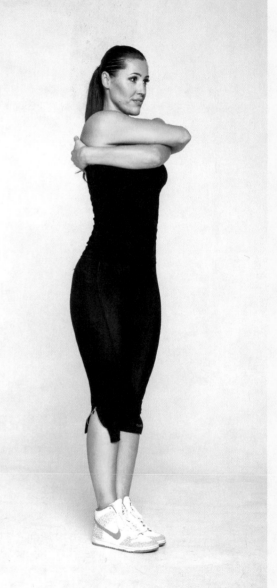

ARM HUGS

Stand upright with your feet together. Bring your arms out to your sides and as far back as you can reach. Bring your arms back to your front, enveloping yourself in a hug.

- 1 x 12
- **Warms up:** Chest and shoulders.

78 BUILDING

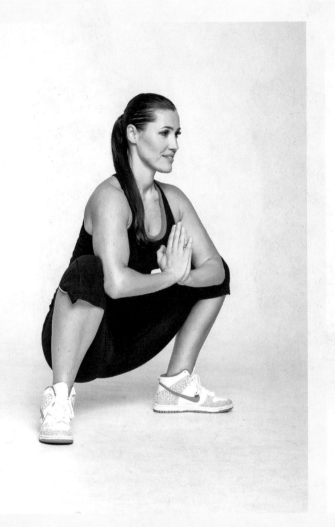

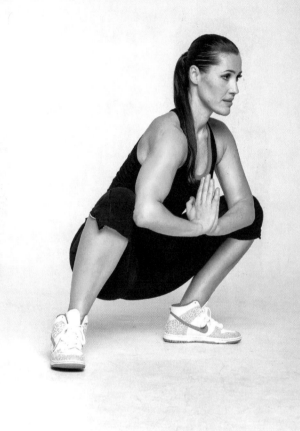

YOGA SQUAT

Stand with your feet wide apart, toes pointing out. Go into a deep squat and try to sit there as comfortably as possible. Place your upper arms inside your knees, keeping your back straight and palms together. Push the legs apart with your arms, while swinging gently from side to side at the same time.

- 1 x 20 swings
- **Warms up:** Lumbar region, groin, and hips.

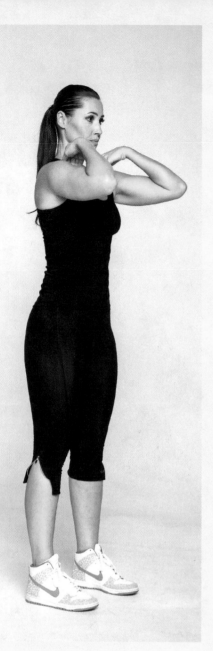
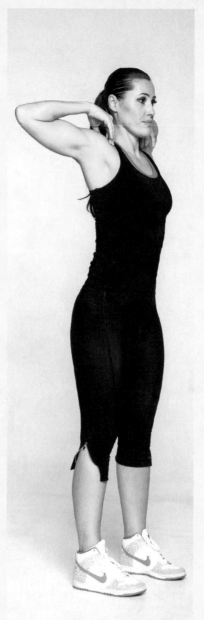
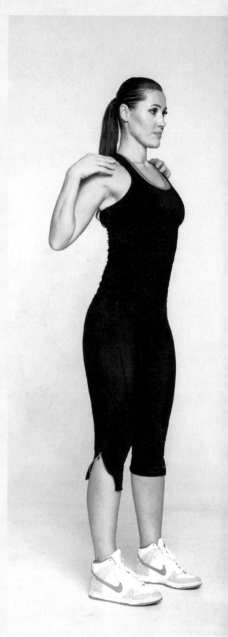

SHOULDER ROLL

Stand upright with your feet shoulder-width apart.
Place your hands on your shoulders. Make large circles
with your arms, first going backward, then forward.

• 1 x 10 on each side
• **Warms up:** Shoulders.

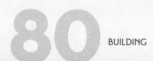

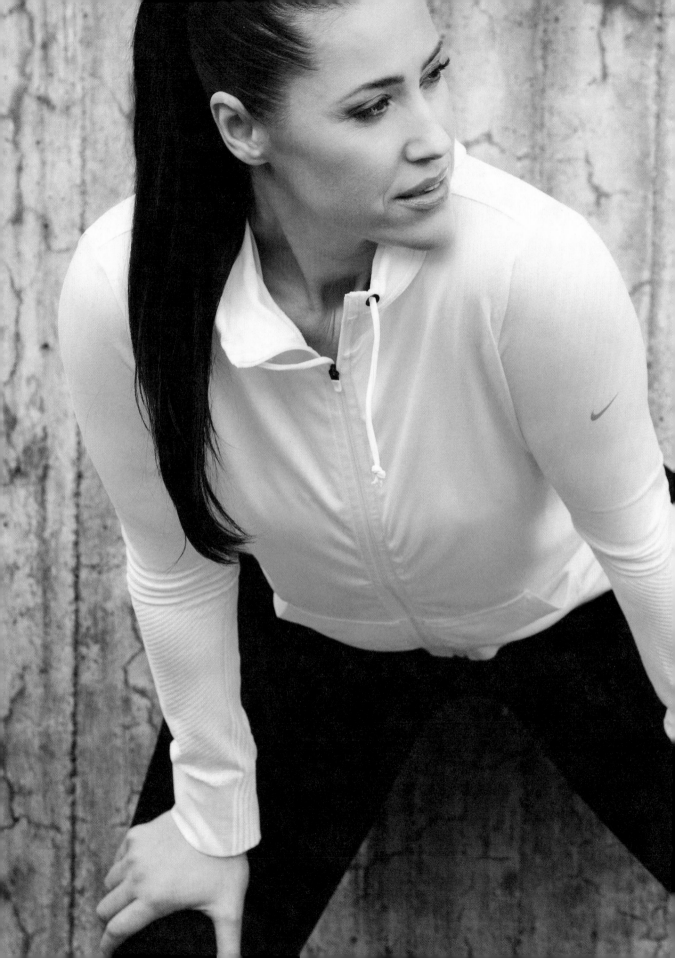

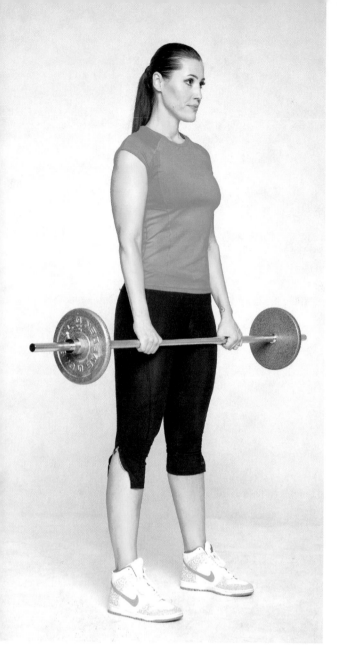

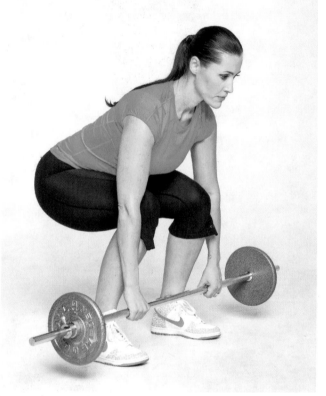

BARBELL DEAD LIFT 1

Stand upright with your feet shoulder-width apart. Grip the barbell firmly with hands shoulder-width apart, with your arms hanging straight down and palms facing you. Lower your hips and bend your knees, moving your hips as far back as possible and bending your torso forward, your back straight but with its natural arch. Keep the barbell close to your body throughout the exercise.

Reverse the steps of this exercise once the barbell hits slightly below the knees. Return to the straight, starting position, and avoid locking your knees.

• **Don't forget:** Keep a natural arch and keep your gaze pointed forward/down toward the floor (if not, you'll strain your neck and shoulders).

• **You're working:** Your glutes, hamstrings, and lower back.

TIP!

• This exercise can also be done with dumbbells.

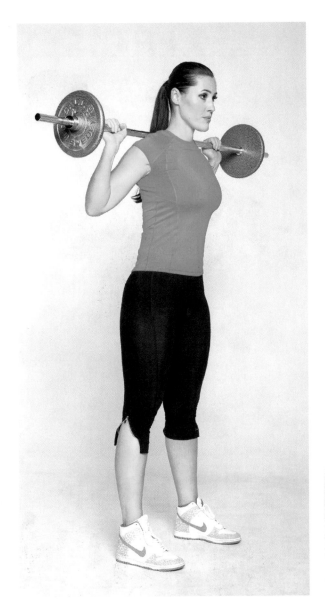

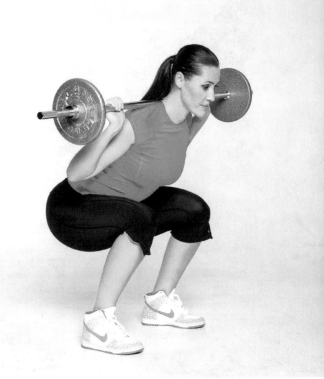

SQUAT WITH A BARBELL

Stand upright with your feet shoulder-width apart. Set a barbell on your shoulders behind your neck, making sure it's not placed directly on the vertebrae. Keep your chest forward and the natural arch in your back. Your knees should be in alignment with your toes.

Now, imagine that you are going to sit down. Move your hips back, and bend your knees to 90 degrees or as deeply as you can manage. Avoid pointing your knees inward as you move up into standing position again.

- **Don't forget:** Avoid rounding your lower back, pointing your knees inward, and working your back instead of your legs.
- **You're working:** Your glutes and legs.

TIP!
- Keep your body weight over your heels but without lifting your toes when you reverse the movement. Maybe place a pair of weighted barbell plates under your heels so you can squat deeper.

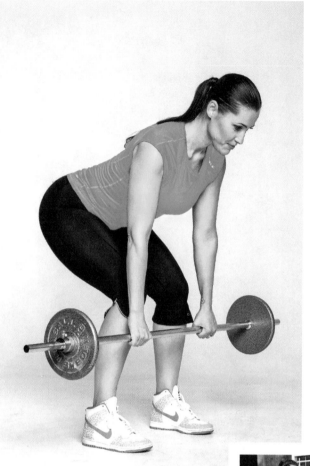

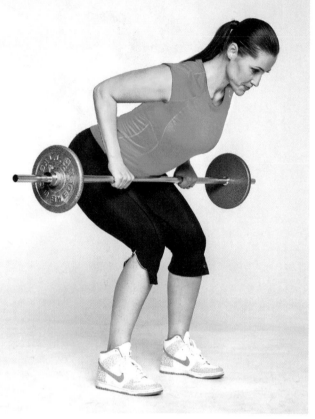

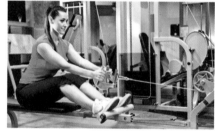

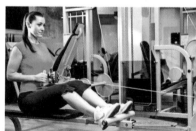

BENT OVER ROW

Stand with lightly bent legs and bring your torso forward. Keep a neutral arch in your back. Grip the barbell a bit wider than shoulder width with palms facing you, keeping your arms straight and chest lifted. Pull the barbell toward your belly, hold, and return to the starting position.

• **Don't forget:** Keep your elbows close to your body. Avoid rounding your lower back and locking your knees.

• **You're working:** Your back and biceps.

TIPS!
• If you're working out in a gym, you can use a rowing machine for this exercise.
• Change your grip occasionally; you can vary it with an underhand grip to allow your biceps to work a little more.

84

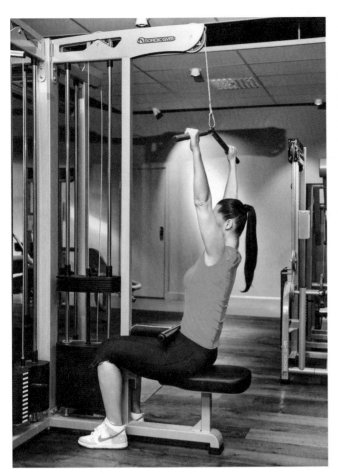

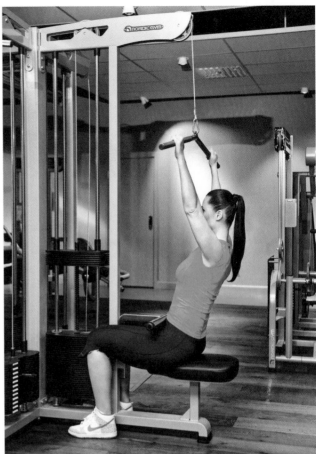

PULL DOWN (BONUS EXERCISE FOR THE GYM)

Sit as close to the machine as you can, with your back leaning slightly backward. Grab the cable's bar with a grip slightly wider than shoulder width, and keep your arms straight.

Lower your shoulders and pull the cable's bar to your chest. Return to straight arms.

• **Don't forget:** Avoid rounding your lower back, and don't pull the cable's bar down first.
• **You're working:** Your back and biceps.

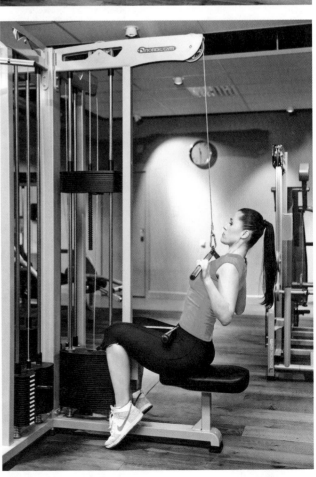

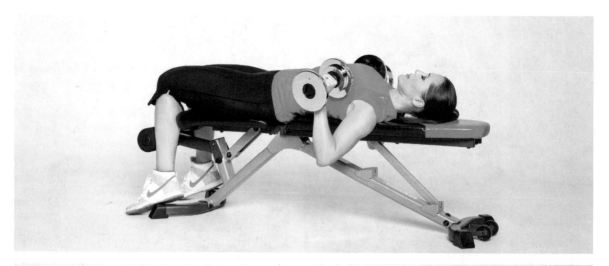

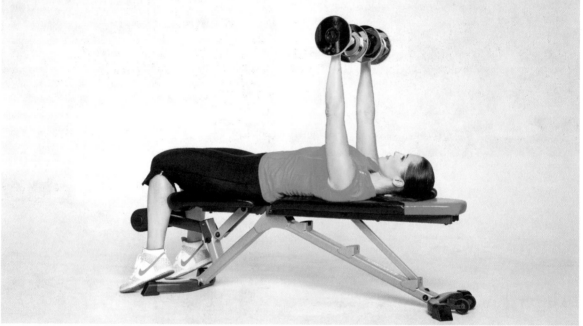

DUMBBELL BENCH PRESS

Lie down on a flat bench and keep your feet on the floor. Hold a pair of dumbbells in your hands, arms bent and positioned close to the side of your chest. Push the dumbbells toward the ceiling until your arms are almost fully extended. Lower the dumbbells to the starting position.

• **Don't forget:** Avoid rounding your lower back. Keep the dumbbells away from the front of your face.
• **You're working:** Your chest and triceps.

TIPS!
• Vary this exercise by performing it on the floor.
• Use a stability ball instead of a flat bench.

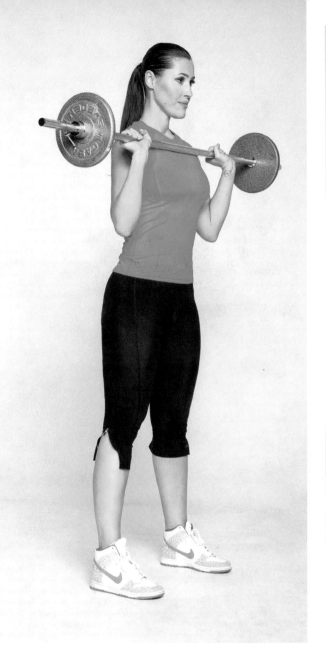

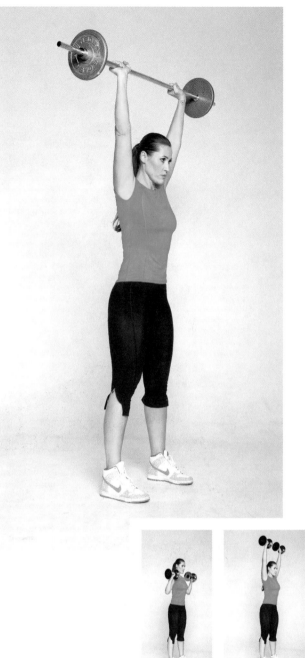

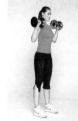

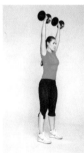

MILITARY SHOULDER PRESS

Stand upright with your feet shoulder-width apart. Hold a barbell with a pronated grip (palms facing forward), your grip slightly wider than shoulder width.

Push the barbell up until your arms are almost fully extended. Lower to the starting position.

- **Don't forget:** Avoid rounding your lower back and tensing your shoulders.
- **You're training:** Your shoulders.

TIP!
- Vary this exercise by using dumbbells.

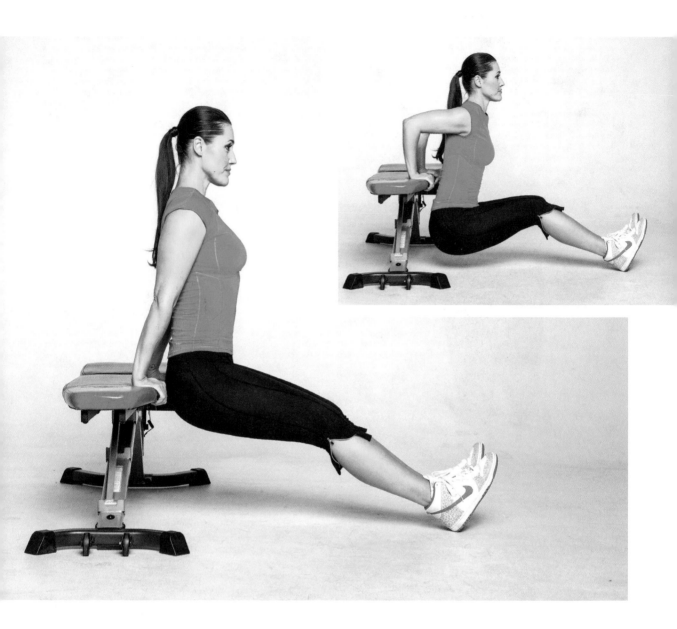

DIPS

Place your hands close behind your back on a flat bench. Keep your back straight and close to the bench. Your feet are on the floor. Bend your arms until your elbows are at a 90-degree angle, and then push back up to the starting position.

• **Don't forget:** Avoid letting your arms spread apart.

• **You're working:** Your triceps and chest.

TIP!
• Make this exercise more challenging by placing weights on your hips.

88

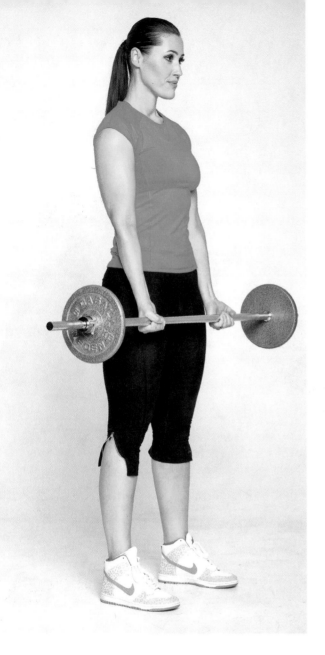

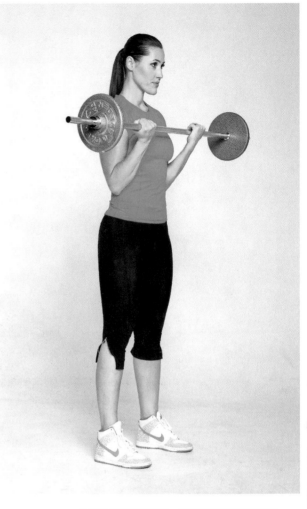

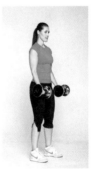
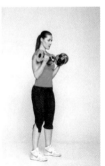

BARBELL BICEPS CURLS

Stand upright without rounding your lower back, and keep your upper arms tight against your body. Grip a barbell with your palms facing you. Keep your elbows somewhat apart from your body and slightly bent.

Lift your forearms toward your chest, hold the position for a moment, and then lower to the starting position. Make sure your wrists are straight and steady.

• **Don't forget:** Avoid rocking your body.
• **You're working:** Your biceps.

TIPS!
• You can do this exercise with dumbbells.
• Vary by switching around your grip to make it pronated (palms away from you).

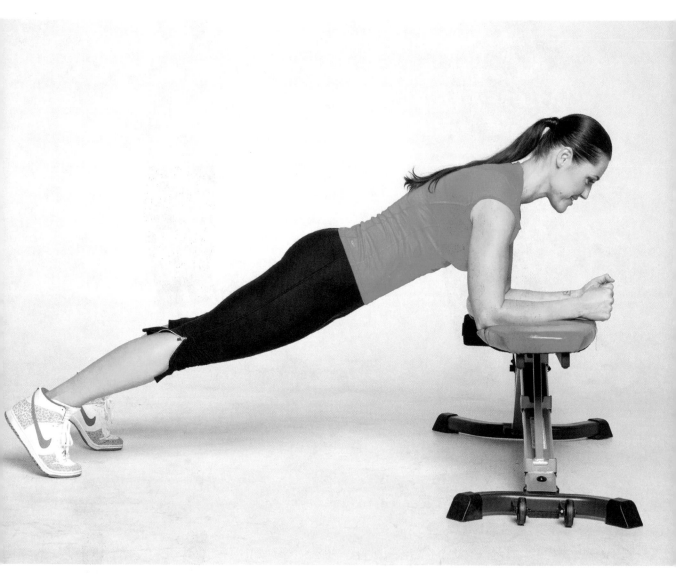

BENCH PLANK

Place your elbows against a bench, keeping your feet shoulder-width apart. Form a straight line with your body, without rounding your lower back, and hold your pelvis in a neutral position.

• **You're working:** Your core, back, shoulders, and front of thighs (quadriceps).

TIP!
• To make the exercise more challenging, move your feet back a few steps and/or lift one leg about 4 inches (10 cm).

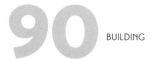

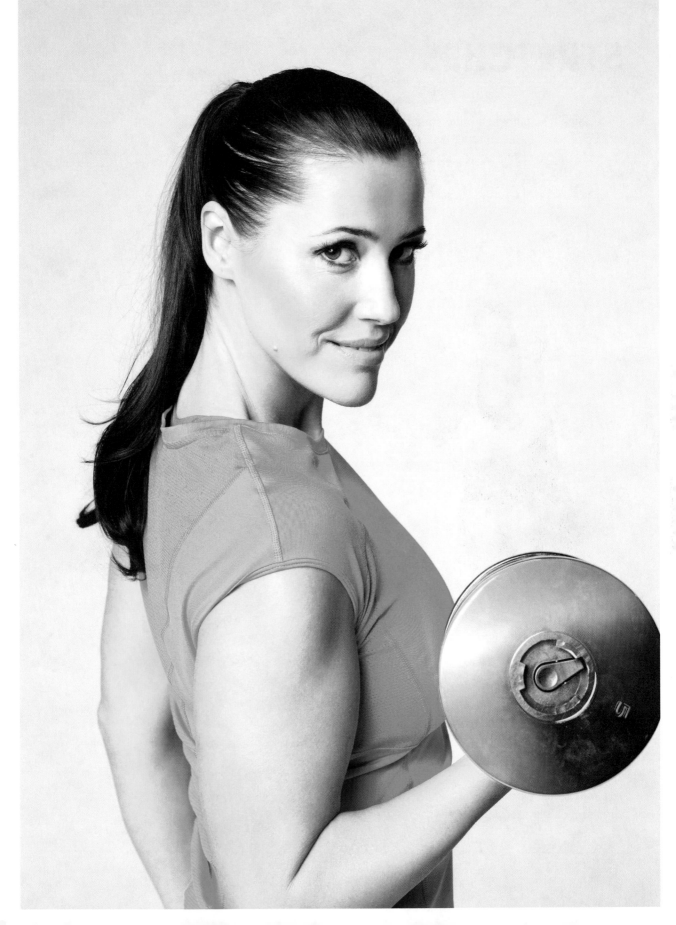

STRETCHES

I like using a stability ball while stretching. It helps soothe the body in a completely different way than if you were doing the exercises standing up; you can also access different angles of the muscles by rolling on the ball.

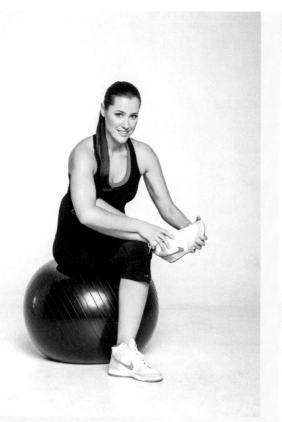

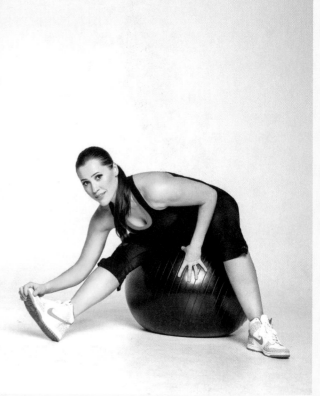

GLUTE STRETCH

Sit on a stability ball. Place one shin on the other leg's knee and lean forward. Increase the stretch by rolling slightly to the right or left on the ball. See which works best.

- 1 x 1 minute per side
- **You're stretching:** Your glutes and lumbar spine.

HAMSTRING STRETCH

Sit on the stability ball, stretch both legs out, and keep them wide apart. Lean forward toward one leg. Keep both legs slightly bent at the knees.

- 1 x 1 minute per side
- **You're stretching:** Your hamstrings.

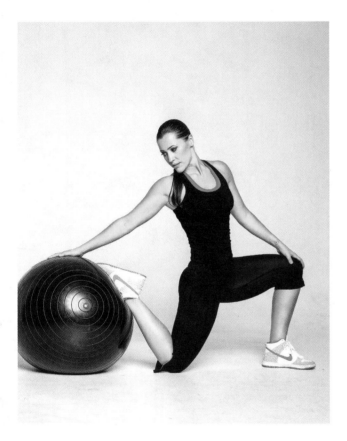

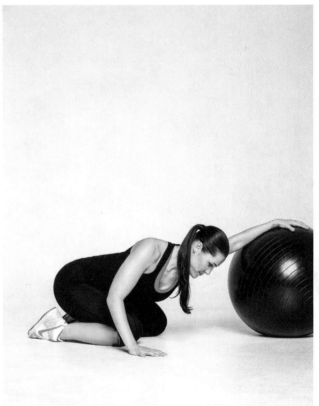

HIP FLEXOR STRETCH

Get down on your knees. Place the top of one foot on the stability ball and position the other leg so your foot rests on the floor. Lower yourself until you feel your hip flexor stretching. Try leaning backward into the ball to increase the stretch.

- 1 x 1 minute per side
- **You're stretching:** Your hip flexors.

CHEST STRETCH

Get on your hands and knees. Place one arm on the stability ball and press your shoulder down toward the floor while at the same time rotating your body slightly out and sideways. Try rolling the ball to stretch different parts of the chest muscle.

- 1 x 1 minute per side.
- **You're stretching:** Your chest and front of shoulder.

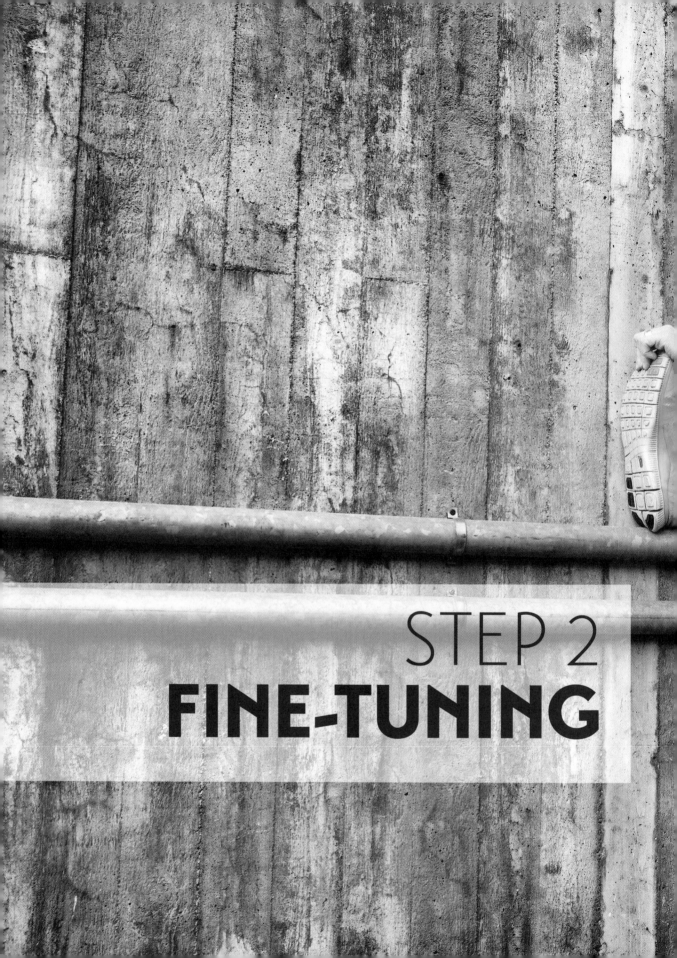

STEP 2
FINE-TUNING

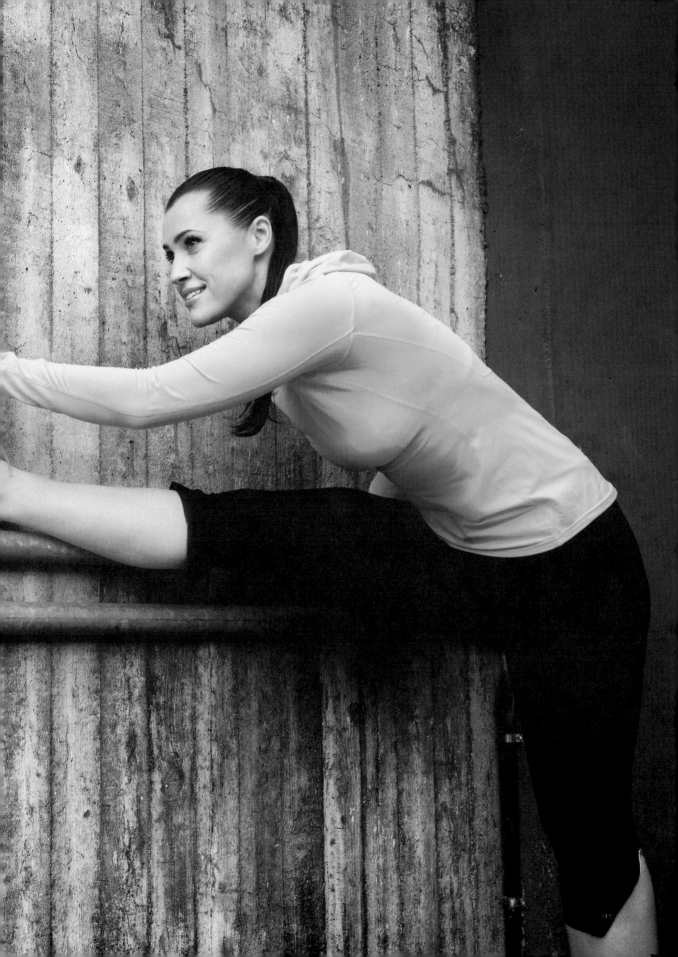

DO YOU SEE ANY IMPROVEMENTS?

The aim of the first and second steps is to build muscle, so weight loss might not happen. Don't forget, we're using up excess calories right now. Concentrate on effort and on improving your strength, not weight loss. Consider it a bonus if the scales tip back and register a loss. When we're rebuilding our body, the scales might stay put even though our body is undergoing changes. Try to observe your progress visually, since the scales are not the best tool for this stage. Instead, compare your current measurements with your "before" pictures. Have they changed since the beginning of the project? Perhaps you're experiencing some of the following improvements already:

- Do you sleep better? Do you wake up feeling rested?
- How's your mood? Are you happier? In a good mood?
- How about PMS? Has it decreased?
- Do you feel stronger in your everyday life?
- Have you stuck with the workouts, even when things were feeling difficult?
- Are you holding your ground at the gym; do you feel like "one of the boys"?

If you don't feel rested and energetic, how's your sleep? Sleep is incredibly important. If you're not rested, you're more likely to make bad decisions and be tempted by cravings. It's easier too to fall into a slump and be negative, and you might also notice that when you're tired you're at greater risk of blowing off a workout and taking to the couch instead. Too little sleep can also increase stress hormones in the blood, which tends to increase feelings of hunger. This in turn can drive you to eat more than you need.

SOME TIPS FOR A BETTER NIGHT'S SLEEP
- Go to bed at a reasonable hour so you get all the sleep you need.
- Sleep in a darkened room.
- Avoid alcohol before going to bed.
- Limit your consumption of coffee in the evening.
- Limit the amount of TV you watch in the evening; turn it off one hour before going to bed.
- Turn off your cell phone before going to bed.

Don't forget your goals. A good way to keep them at the forefront is to write down the reasons why you want to work on your training and your health. Do you want to develop more muscle tone or do you want to feel more energy and stamina? Bring out those reminder notes whenever you find your motivation wavering.

WORKOUT ROUTINE

In the first step we worked hard on large muscles. Now that we have a good, strong base, we will continue the training by targeting the smaller muscles such as the biceps, triceps, and shoulders. Reps are increased, but the emphasis is still on building muscle. Use weights heavy enough that you can only manage 8 repetitions. After a while try for 9, 10, etc., until you can complete 12 repetitions. Once you can do that, increase the weight and start again with 8 repetitions, and continue increasing the reps until you can finish 12.

I build my workout routines around two or three basic exercises per muscle group. Here I've added isolation exercises—exercises that target one specific muscle at a time. These are best done toward the end of the workout, when coordination and balance is beginning to weaken but you still want to work the muscle to failure. Hip thrusts and French presses are two examples of isolation exercises in this routine. Two similar exercises for the same muscle can affect the muscle differently. For example, in this routine you'll do standing biceps curls and seated biceps curls on an incline bench (pages 102, 113). Even though there are similarities between those exercises, the movements are in fact very different and will challenge the muscle in distinct ways.

In this step we'll also be using the "split training" system. This means you will be working on two to three muscle groups/body parts per day, working them until total fatigue, and then letting them recover for a few days. With this method, muscles get worked about twice a week and have 48 to 72 hours' rest, which gives them enough time to recover and handle the next workout.

In this step you'll do both low and high intensity cardio exercises (HIIT— read more about it on page 98), which is to be performed after a rest day and before the leg workout on Mondays. This leaves you with enough strength to give it your all.

New in this step is the superset, which consists of two exercises performed one right after the other, with no rest in between. You go through the first exercise and move straight on to the second. Then you rest, and repeat the sequence again, a certain amount of times. (See the workout routine on page 133.)

The exercises begin on page 100. You'll find three different workout routines as well as a weekly schedule on pages 133 to 136.

HOW LONG DOES THIS STEP LAST?

I recommend that the fine-tuning step take place over eight weeks. This step features a lot of variety, so the entire body gets to work.

CARDIO FOR STEP 2

I have planned both low and high intensity cardio workouts for the week. You can perform high intensity cardio in several ways, but I prefer HIIT (read more about HIIT on page 27). Here are two different routines you can do in rotation.

Remember not to start out too fast or too hard; get the feel for the workout first. How much can you handle? How does it feel? Where do you feel it? If you do interval running on a treadmill, it's imperative that you move your arms properly and pay attention to how your core works, because everything works together.

HIIT 1

This workout can be done on your choice of indoor cardio equipment, or outside.
It will take 15 to 20 minutes (not including warm-up and cool-down). Start by doing 10 minutes for a few weeks, then increase it to 15 minutes, and end with 20 minutes after 4 to 5 weeks.

Warm-up: Jog, or cycle, for 5 minutes.
Run/bike as fast as you can for 30 seconds, and then revert back to active rest for 90 seconds (jog lightly, walk, or bike slowly to bring down your heart rate).
• Repeat 10 to 12 times.
Cool-down: Walk or bike at low speed for 5 minutes.

HIIT 2

This workout can be performed on your choice of indoor cardio equipment, or outside.
Perform 5- to 8-minute workouts for a few weeks (not including warm-up and cool-down), and then increase your time little by little to a total of 20 minutes.

Warm-up: Jog or cycle for 5 minutes.
Run/bike as fast as you can for 20 seconds, then rest for 40 seconds (you can hop off the treadmill, but don't forget to hold onto the handles as you do this), walking slowly or biking slowly to lower your heart rate.
• Repeat 15 times.
Cool-down: Walk or bike at low speed for 5 minutes.

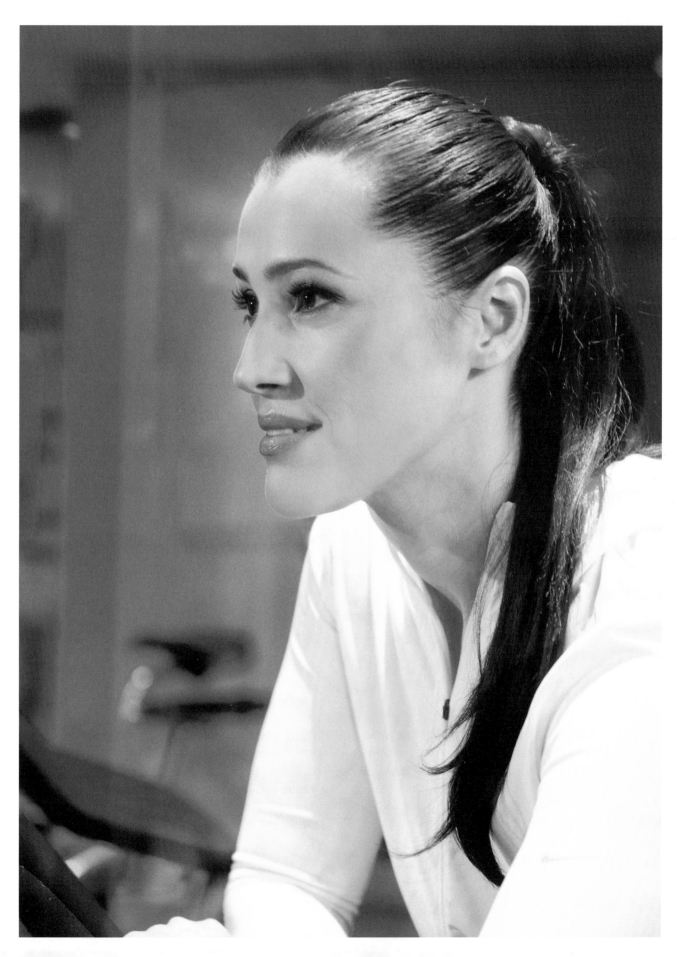

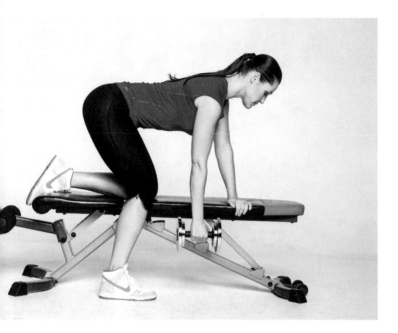

EXERCISES

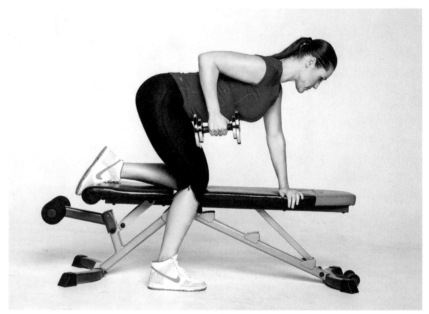

ONE ARM ROW

Lean forward and place one arm and one knee on a flat bench. Pull a dumbbell up the side of your body by lifting your elbow as far back as you can.

• **Don't forget:** Avoid rotating your body. Make sure that your elbow stays near your body when you pull your elbow back.
• **You're working:** Your back and biceps.

TIP!
• You can use a chair instead of a flat bench.

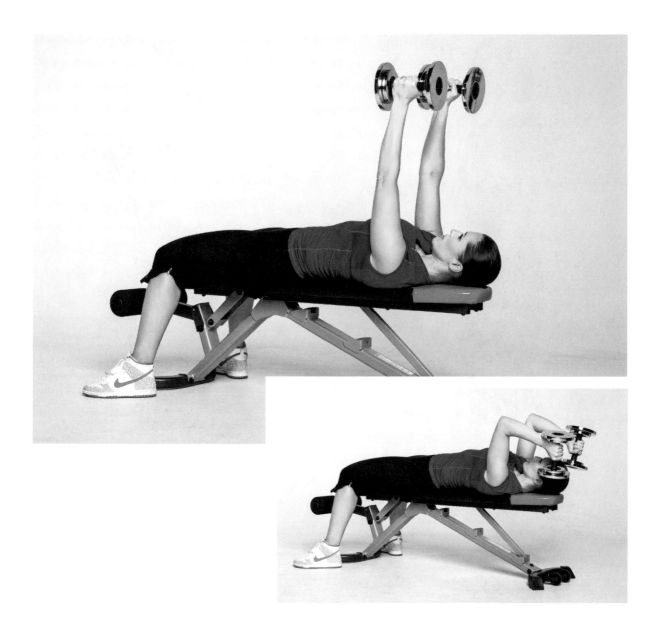

FRENCH PRESS WITH DUMBBELLS

Lie down on a flat bench. Hold two dumbbells shoulder-width apart. Extend your arms toward the ceiling. Lower the dumbbells toward your forehead, and return to the starting point.

• **Don't forget:** Keep your arms parallel, and don't spread your elbows when you bring the dumbbells back from the lowered position.
• **You're working:** Your triceps.

TIPS!
• You can lie on the floor with your knees bent instead of using a bench.
• Vary this exercise by doing one side at a time.

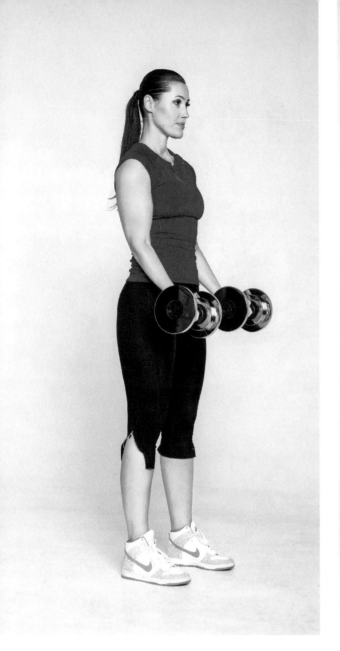
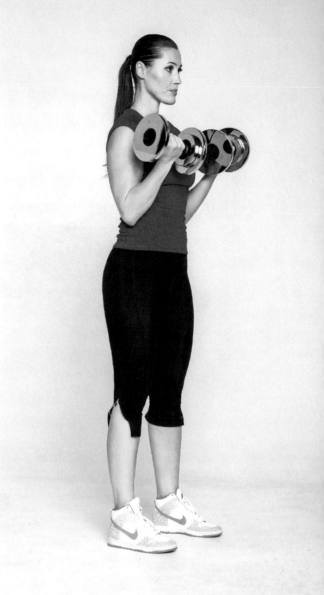

DUMBBELL BICEPS CURLS

Stand upright, with your feet about shoulder-width apart. Hold the dumbbells at shoulder width, palms facing you. Keep your elbows tight against your sides. Lift the dumbbells by bending your elbows. Return to the starting position.

• **Don't forget:** Keep your upper arms close to your body. Avoid rocking your body.
• **You're working:** Your biceps.

TIPS!
• This exercise works well with a barbell, too.
• Vary this exercise by using a pronated grip.

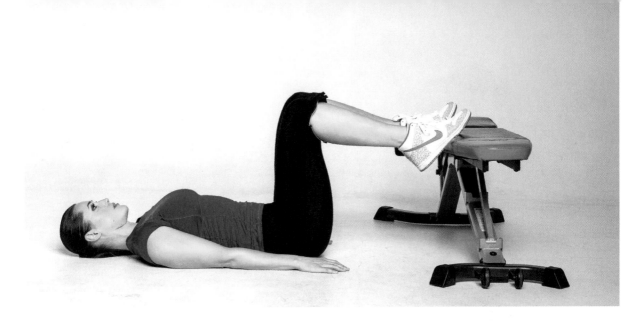

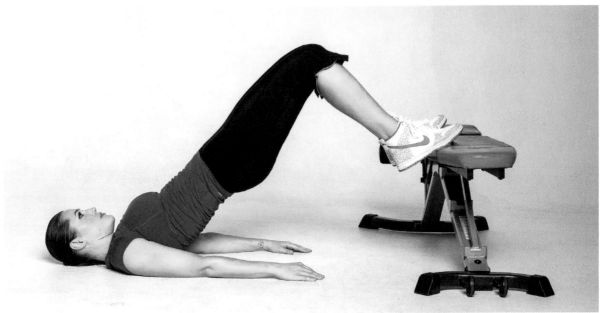

GLUTE BRIDGE

Lie flat on your back, with feet about shoulder-width apart and on a bench. Lift your body to make a straight line. Slowly lower it and return to the starting point.

- **Don't forget:** Squeeze your glutes when you're at the top of the movement.
- **You're working:** Your glutes.

TIPS!
- You can put your feet on a chair propped against a wall if you don't have a bench.
- Vary this exercise by doing one side at a time.
- After two weeks, place a weighted plate on your hips (keep it in place with your hands).

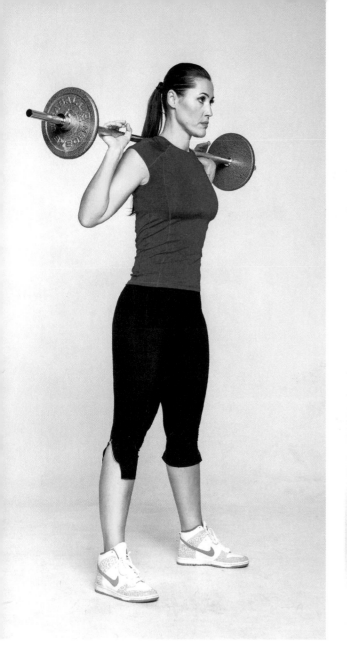
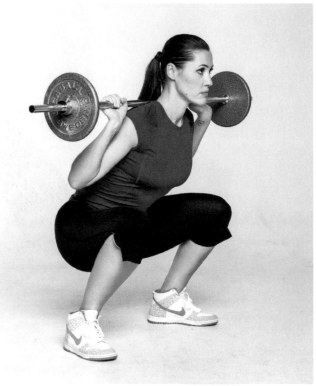

BARBELL DEEP SQUAT

Stand upright with your feet shoulder-width apart and your back in a neutral position. The barbell is placed behind your neck. Hold the barbell with both hands.

Fix your gaze straight ahead and squat down as far as you're able. Return to the starting position.

• **Don't forget:** Your form; avoid rounding your back. Your knees should align with your toes; don't turn them inward on the way up.
• **You're working:** Your glutes, legs, and back.

TIP!
• Place a pair of weighted plates or books under your heels if you have difficulty squatting.

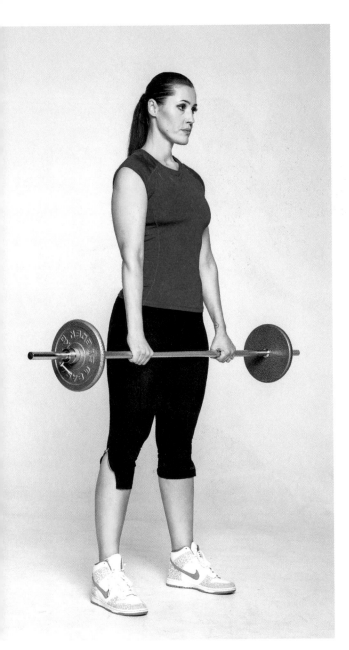
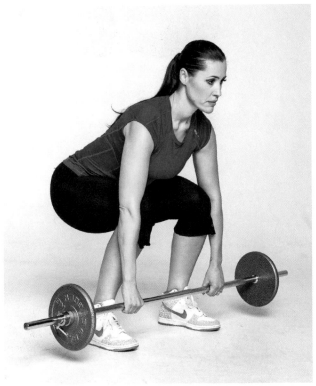

DEAD LIFT

Stand with your feet shoulder-width apart and arms straight, and firmly hold the barbell in front of your body.

Bend at the knees, bringing your hips as far back as possible and bending your torso forward, your back straight but with a neutral arch. When the barbell hits just below the knees, return to your starting upright stance but avoid locking your knees. Count to 1 on the way down, and 2–3 when coming back up.

• **Don't forget:** Keep the barbell close to your body at all times.
• **You're working:** Your glutes, hamstrings, and back.

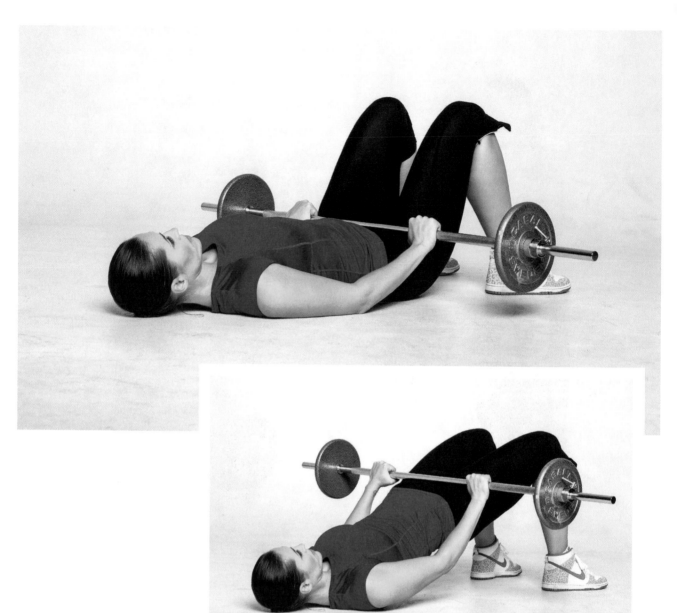

HIP THRUST

Lie on your back, with your feet on the floor about shoulder-width apart. Place a barbell on your hips. Lift your body so it makes a straight line. Squeeze your glutes and hold for 1 second. Slowly return to the starting position.

- **Don't forget:** Knees and feet should be aligned.
- **You're working:** Your glutes.

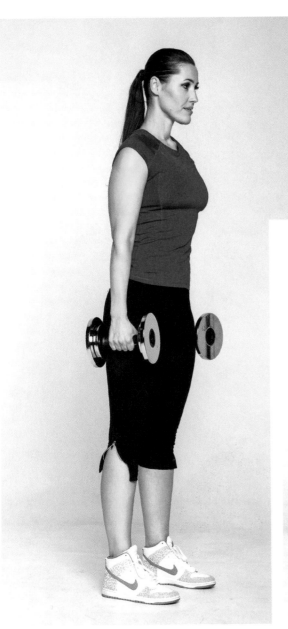

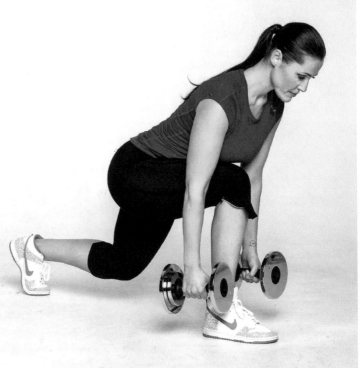

INCLINE REVERSE LUNGE

Stand upright, your feet about shoulder-width apart. Hold on to a pair of dumbbells.

Take one step back, leaning forward and touching the floor with the dumbbells. Return to the starting position.

- **Don't forget:** Don't use dumbbells that are too heavy. Your step is supposed to be long. Keep your back straight throughout the exercise.
- **You're working:** Your glutes, legs, and back.

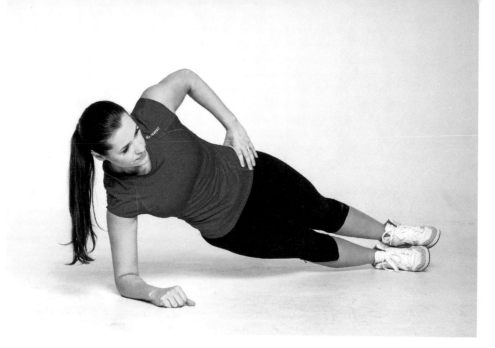

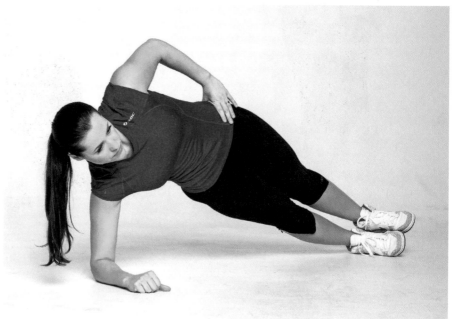

SIDE HIP RAISES

Keep one elbow and forearm on the mat, with your
feet together and your body straight.
    Do small lifts by raising your body toward the ceiling.

• **Don't forget:** Don't rush—control your lifts, and
always return to a proper side plank position.
• **You're working:** Your core muscles.

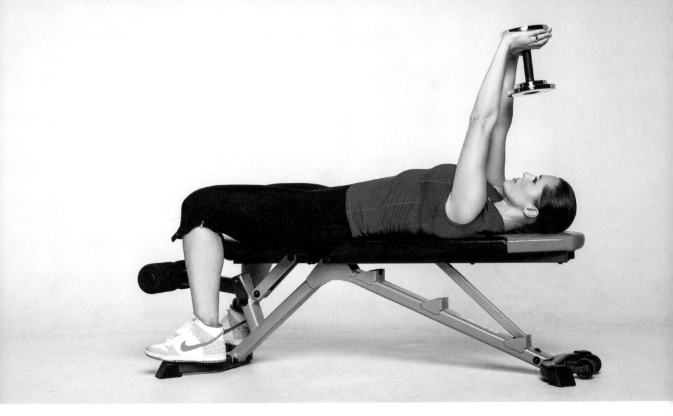

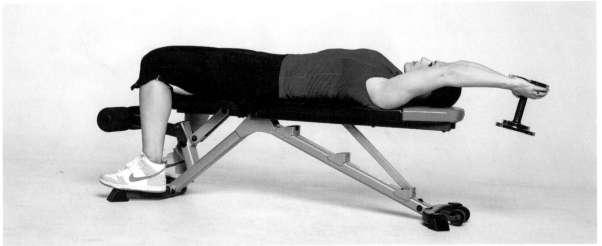

PULLOVER

Lie on your back on a flat bench, and hold on to one dumbbell with both hands. Keep the arms extended toward the ceiling.

Keeping your arms straight, lower the dumbbell behind your head, and stop when you're level with your head. Return to the starting position.

- **Don't forget:** Keep your arms straight, and avoid brushing past your ears with your arms.
- **You're working:** Your back and chest.

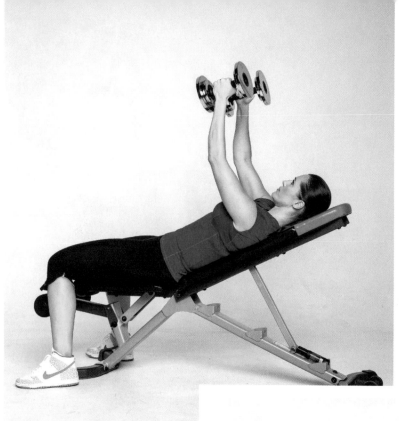

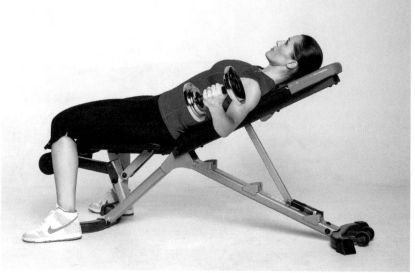

INCLINE DUMBBELL FLIES

Raise your bench to an angle of about 15 degrees. Lie on your back, arms slightly bent out, and hold on to a pair of dumbbells at chest level. Bring the dumbbells up in an arch over your chest (not over your face!). Return to the starting position.

- **Don't forget:** Avoid bending you arms too much.
- **You're working:** Your chest.

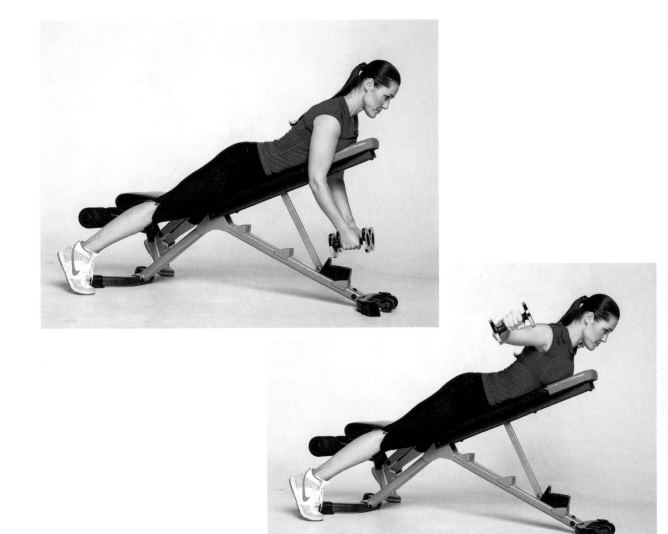

INCLINE REVERSE FLIES

Lie on the inclined bench, your legs straight and and your back in a neutral position. Grab a pair of dumbbells and let your arms hang freely toward the floor.

Move your arms up backward to shoulder level and squeeze your shoulder blades together. Slowly return to the starting position.

- **Don't forget:** Avoid bending your arms too much. Keep your back in a neutral position.
- **You're working:** Your posterior shoulder.

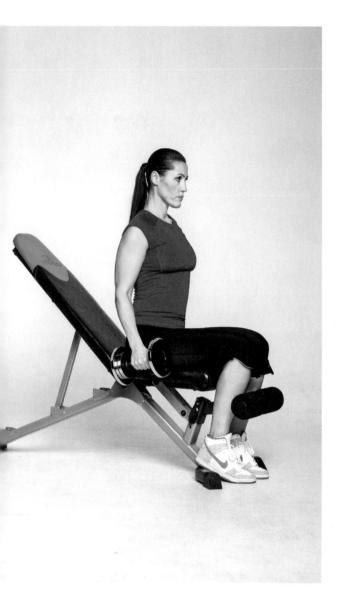
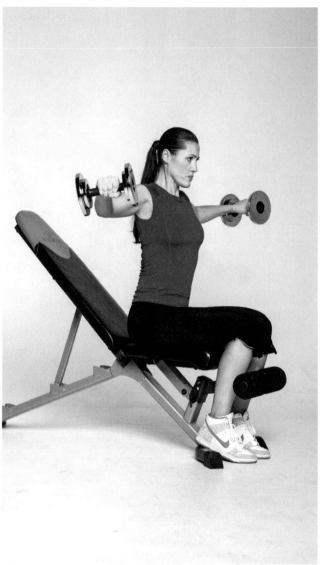

SEATED SIDE LATERAL RAISE

Sit up straight on a bench. Hold a dumbbell in each hand, arms straight down at your sides.

Keeping your elbows slightly bent, lift the dumbbells up laterally to about shoulder level. Return slowly to starting position.

- **Don't forget:** Avoid bending your arms and tensing your neck.
- **You're working:** Your shoulders.

TIP!
- Vary this exercise by alternating arms.

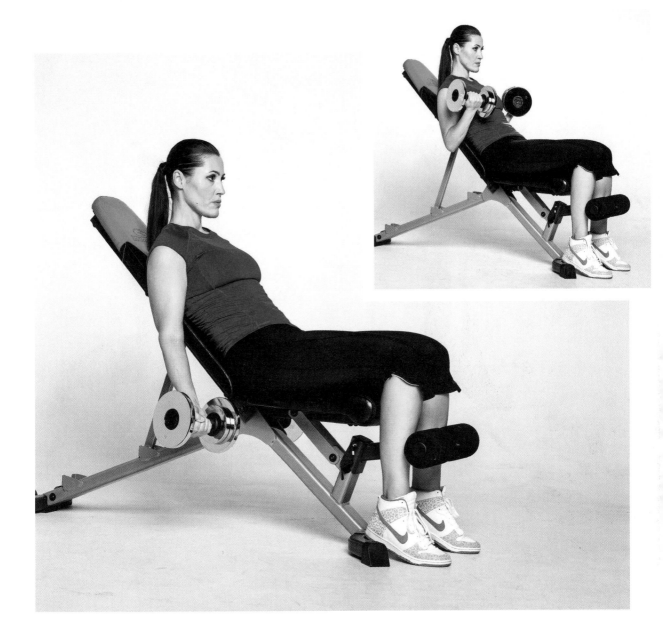

INCLINE DUMBBELL CURLS

Lean back against the bench's back support, arms hanging straight down with elbows slightly bent. Hold the dumbbells with your palms facing you. Lift your lower arms up toward you, squeeze, and lower the dumbbells to the starting position. Make sure that your wrists are straight and steady.

- **Don't forget:** Avoid rocking your body.
- **You're working:** Your biceps.

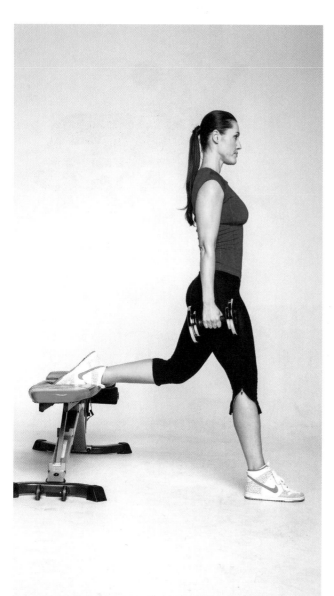
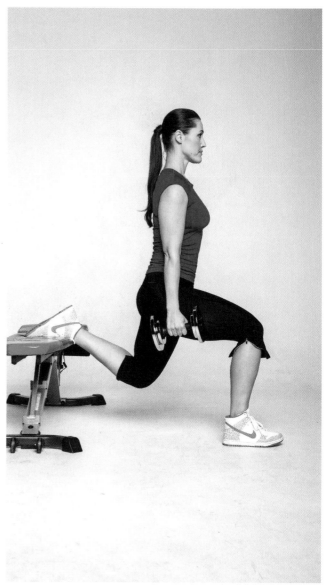

BULGARIAN SPLIT SQUAT

Stand upright with the top of one foot on the bench. Hold on to a pair of dumbbells. Lower your body into a squat, and slowly straighten up to the starting position.

• **Don't forget:** Keep your back straight. Be careful where you put your body weight; make your glutes work.

• **You're working:** Your glutes and legs.

TIP!
• You can lean a chair against the wall instead of using a bench.

114

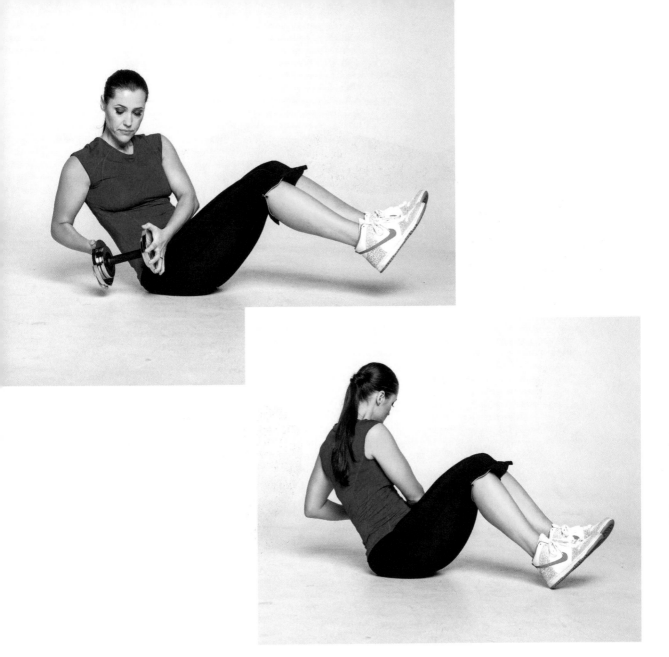

RUSSIAN TWIST

Sit on the floor with your back in a neutral position. Keep your legs slightly bent and hold a dumbbell with both hands.

From your trunk, start turning the dumbbell from side to side.

- **Don't forget:** Keep your back long and straight.
- **You're working:** Your core muscles.

TIP!
- If too difficult, perform the exercise with your feet resting on the floor.

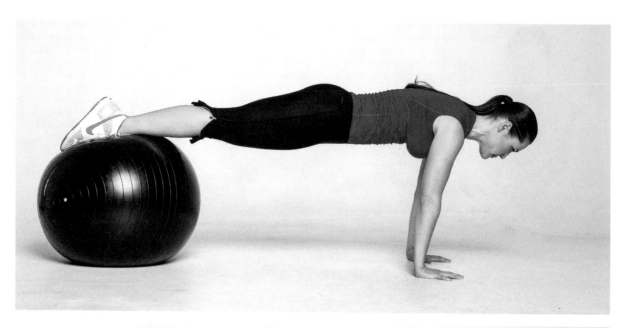

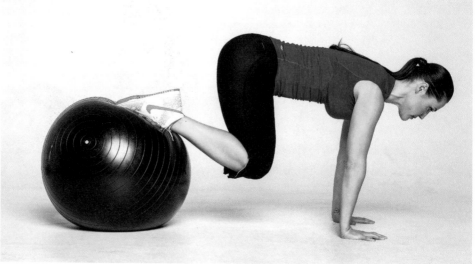

STABILITY BALL KNEE TUCK-IN

Place your feet on a stability ball and your hands flat on the floor under your shoulders. Put your body into a plank, with your back in a neutral position.

With your feet, pull the ball in toward you, and then return it to the starting position.

• **Don't forget:** Avoid swaying your back and dropping your shoulders.
• **You're working:** Your core muscles and shoulders.

TIP!
• To make the exercise more challenging, place only your toes on the ball.

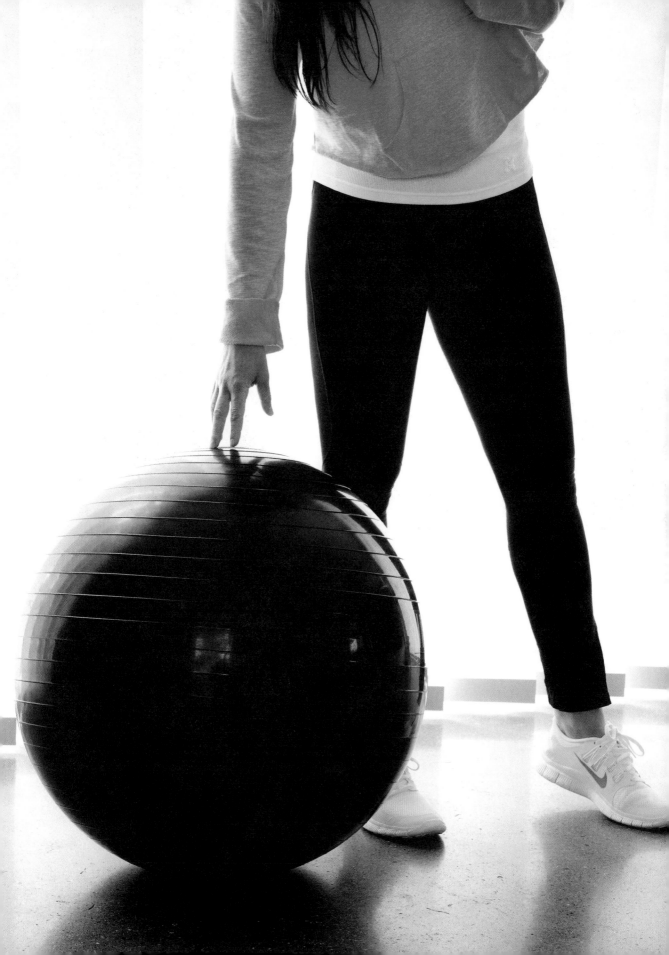

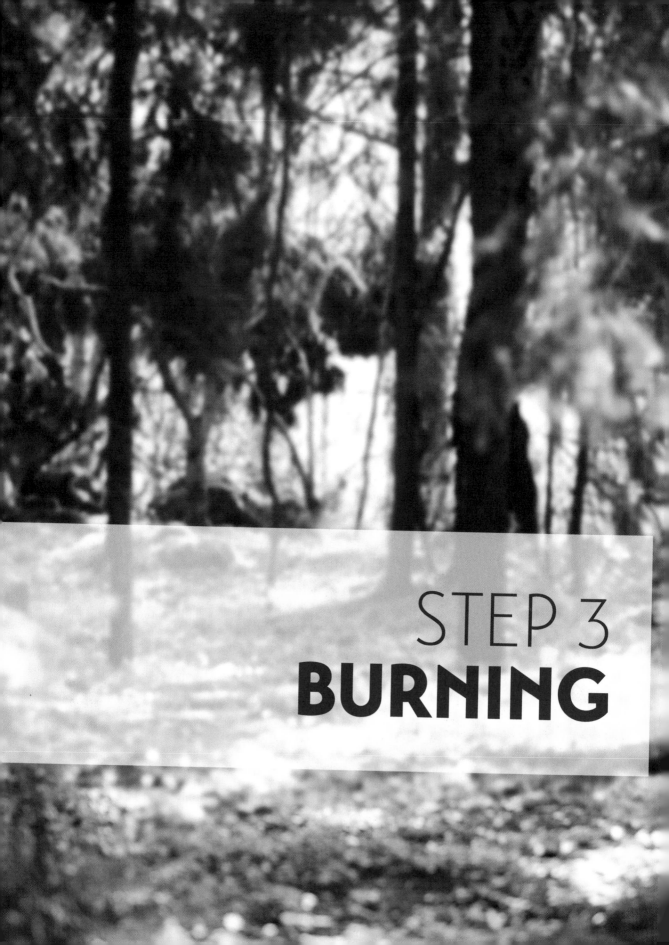

STEP 3
BURNING

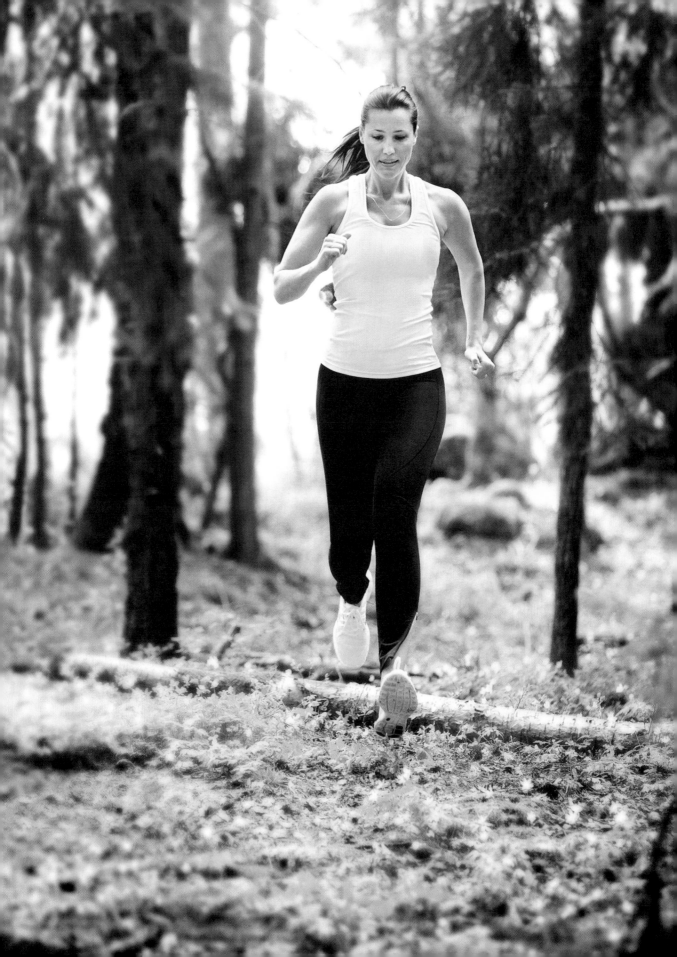

SHOW OFF THOSE MUSCLES!

We've made it to the fun bit—the muscles you've built are now about to be displayed. This is so exciting!

One problem that might emerge at this stage is you could want to start treating yourself to things that were "forbidden" before. You might be experiencing the feeling that you've sacrificed or missed something. Stop right now! Think about it. There will always be events to celebrate—Christmas, New Year, Easter, Mardi Gras, school graduations, music festivals, cozy Fridays, and vacations. All these special occasions are commemorated with food—candy, cake, sweet rolls, and chips. Are we going to be tempted by all this and start overindulging? No way.

You can be proactive in maintaining your food habits. You can choose to be pleased with your choices and be truly proud of not being swayed by what everyone else is doing. Did you know that eating junk food is considered the norm today rather than the other way around?

Do you remember the note you wrote that stated what you wished to accomplish with your training? Look at it and remind yourself of why you're doing this. Don't forget that you will get stronger psychologically. You might have more stamina, greater patience, and higher self-esteem.

WORKOUT ROUTINE

Things are going to get seriously intense now! This step consists of strength training three times a week, including one day of circuit training, two days of HIIT training, and the remaining days devoted to low intensity cardio workouts—enough to keep your body on high alert and prevent it from getting used to a single routine and the same old weights.

Circuit training targets large muscle groups (mostly with basic exercises) and is strenuous because the rest period between each exercise is very brief. This workout not only burns calories but also has a positive impact on the hormonal system due to the after-burn effect. It's very important that you strive for good form while performing the exercises, and, of course, don't forget to adjust the weights so you don't use the same throughout the workout.

HOW LONG DOES THIS STEP LAST?

Keep it up for eight weeks—or until you are satisfied! (Read more about what you can do as a follow-up on page 140.)

CARDIO FOR STEP 3

Now we're going to optimize our cardio workouts by combining what we've done up until now. Here are two variations on HIIT.

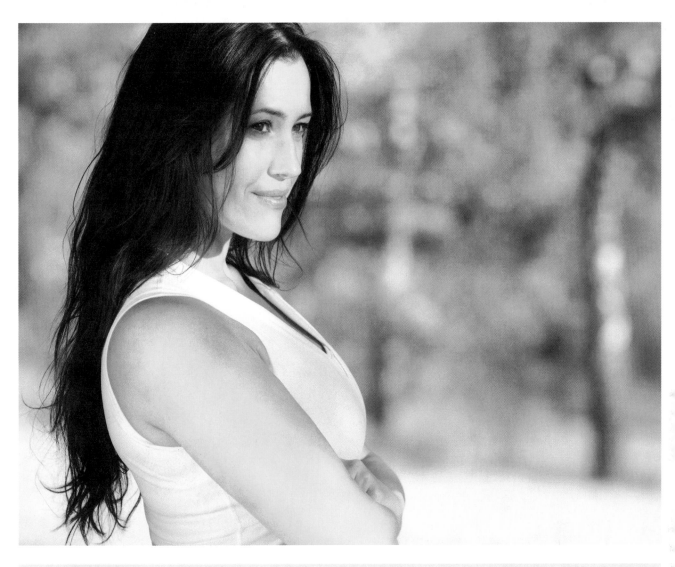

HIIT 1

Warm-up: Lightly jog or walk for 5 minutes.

Run as fast as you can for 30 seconds, then switch to active rest for 90 seconds. Hop off the treadmill at this point if you're using one.

• Repeat for a maximum of 10 times.

Immediately afterward: Low intensity cardio for 30 minutes.

HIIT 2

Warm-up: Lightly jog or walk for 5 minutes.

Run as fast as you can for 10 seconds, then switch to active rest for 50 seconds. Hop off the treadmill at this point if you're using one.

• Repeat for a maximum of 10 times.

Immediately afterward: Low intensity cardio for 30 minutes.

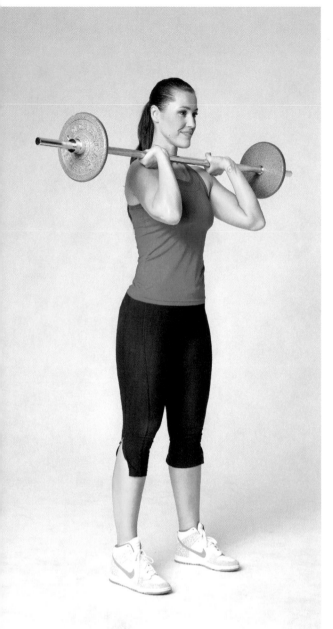

EXERCISES

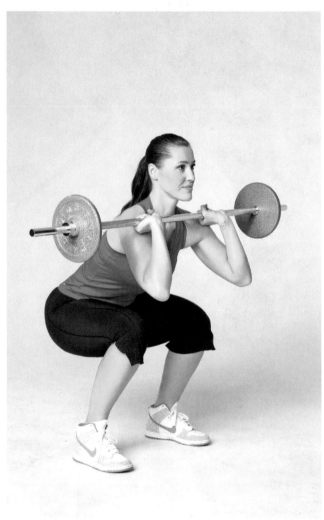

FRONT SQUAT

Stand upright, with your feet shoulder-width apart and your back in neutral position. Hold a barbell, letting the bar rest on top of your deltoids. Push your elbows up so they're level with your shoulders. Look straight ahead and squat as far down as you can. Return to the starting position.

• **Don't forget:** Try to keep your back neutral throughout the entire exercise, and avoid rounding your back. Keep a tight rein on your knees so they don't splay when you're coming back up.
• **You're working:** Your glutes and legs.

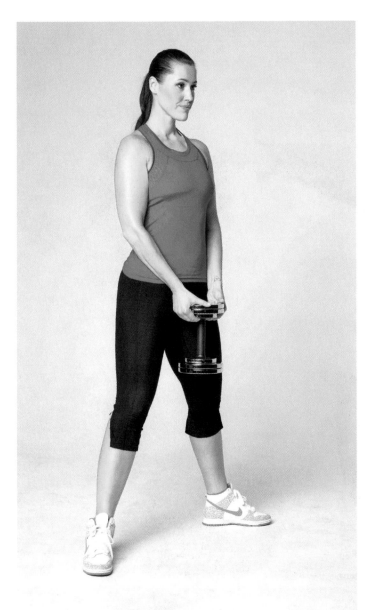

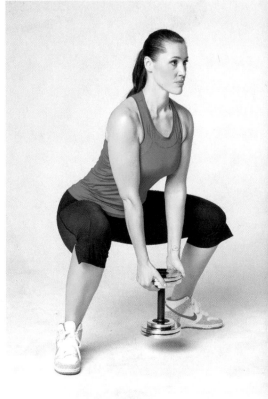

WIDE-STANCE DUMBBELL SQUAT

Stand with your legs wider than shoulder width, your toes pointing out. Your back should be straight and in a neutral position. Grab a dumbbell with both hands and let it hang toward the floor.

Squat as far down as your flexibility allows without letting your knees splay out. Return to the starting position without locking your knees. Squeeze your glutes.

- **Don't forget:** Avoid rounding your back and dropping your torso—think *escalator*, which goes up and down.
- **You're working:** Your glutes and legs.

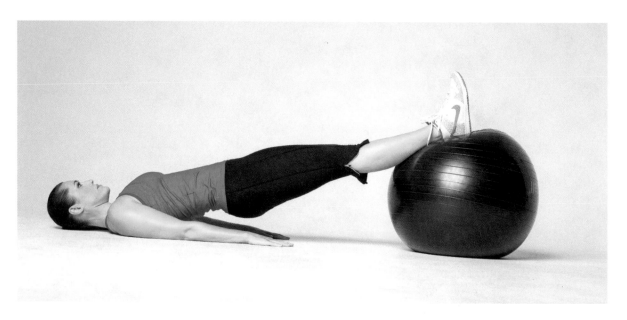

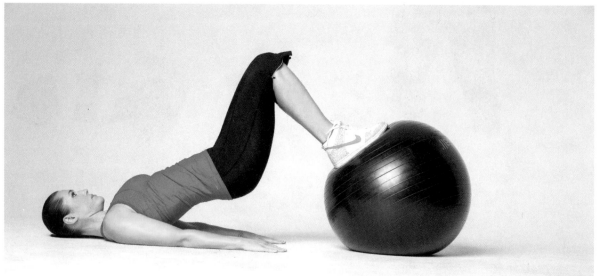

STABILITY BALL HIP ROLL

Lie with calves and feet balanced on top of a stability ball. Raise your pelvis. Your arms should be on the floor and aligned with your body.

Tense the hamstrings on the back of your thighs, and pull the ball toward you with your feet. Roll the ball back to the starting position.

• **Don't forget:** Keep your buttocks elevated throughout the entire exercise.
• **You're working:** Your hamstrings and glutes.

TIP!

• Make this exercise more challenging by lifting your arms off the floor.

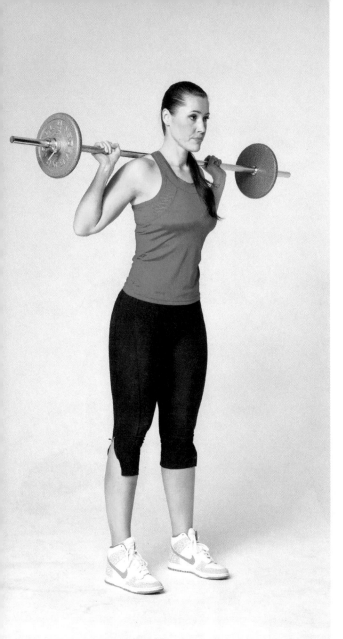

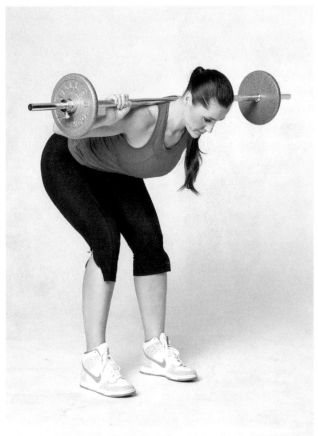

GOOD MORNINGS

Grab a barbell and let it rest just below your neck. Brace your abs and avoid rounding your back; keep your knees slightly bent.

Push your hips back as far as possible and bend your torso forward to make a 90-degree angle. Let your gaze follow as you go. Return to starting position by pushing your hips forward and squeezing your glutes.

• **You're working:** Your glutes and hamstrings.

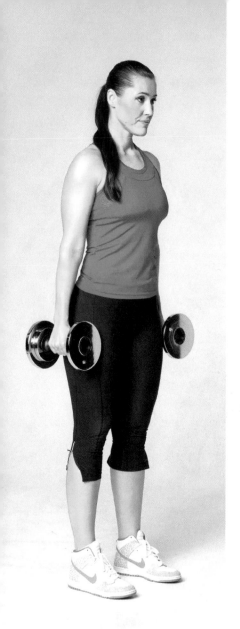
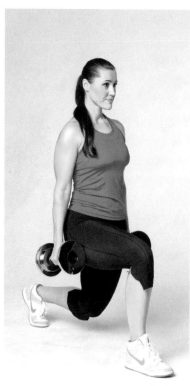
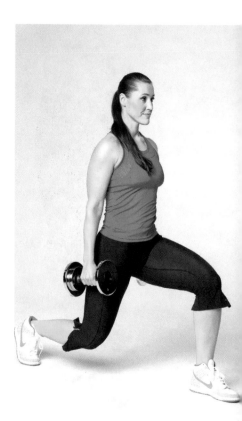

WALKING LUNGE WITH DUMBBELLS

Stand with your feet hip-width apart, and grab a pair of dumbbells.

Using one leg, take one big step forward and sink down toward the floor by bending your knees. Make sure that your knees are aligned with your toes and that your knees don't push past your toes.

• **Don't forget:** Avoid leaning forward; remember that your knees should point in the same direction as your toes.

• **You're working:** Your glutes and legs.

TIP!
• Vary this exercise by using a barbell on your shoulders.

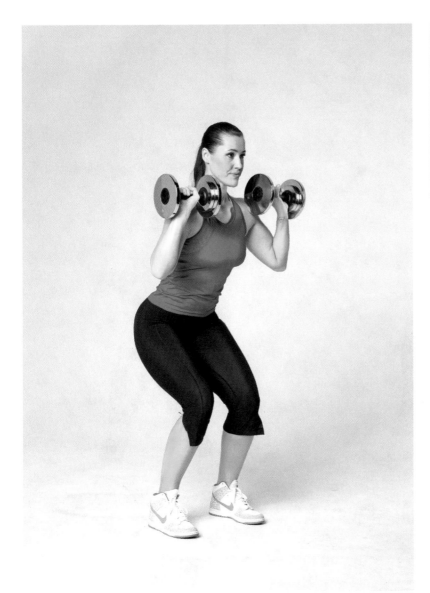
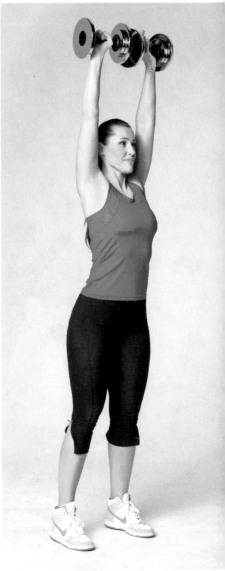

PUSH PRESS WITH DUMBBELLS

Stand with your feet shoulder-width apart and hold a pair of dumbbells level with your ears.

Bend your knees into a mini-squat and then push the dumbbells upward with your whole body.

• **You're working:** Your shoulders and torso.

TIPS!
• Vary this exercise by using a barbell.
• After a few weeks, perform this exercise one arm at a time.

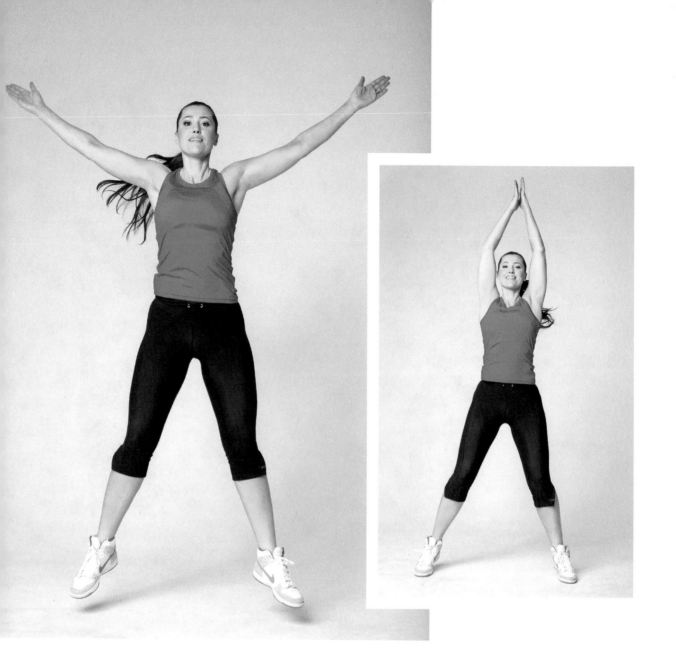

JUMPING JACKS

Stand upright with your feet shoulder-width apart.
  Jump and bring your legs out to the sides so that your feet are wider than shoulder-width apart. Simultaneously, raise your arms over your head. Jump back to the starting position.

• **You're working:** Your general fitness/cardio system.

128 BURNING

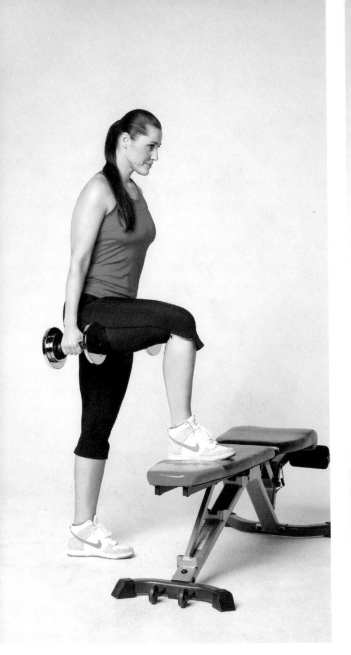
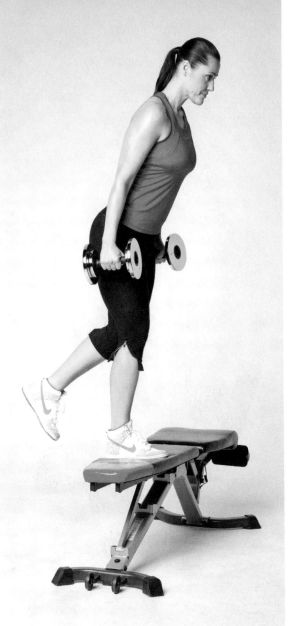

STEP UPS WITH DUMBBELLS

Stand upright with your feet shoulder-width apart. Grab a pair of dumbbells.

Place one foot on a flat bench and step up on to the bench. Keep the weight on that same leg, and step down slowly. Change legs and repeat on the other side.

- **Don't forget:** Keep your body upright or slightly bent forward.

- **You're working:** Your glutes and legs.

TIPS!
- You can use a chair up against a wall instead of a bench.
- Vary this exercise by starting standing on the bench: Take one step down and then step up again.

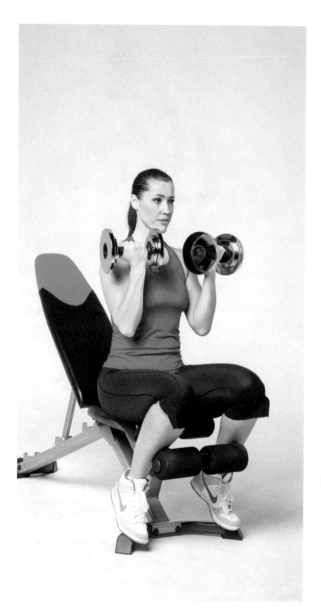
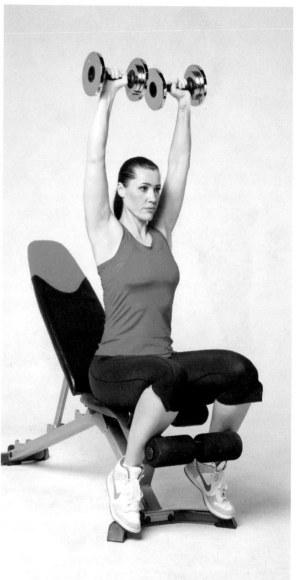

ARNOLD PRESS

Sit on a bench and keep your back straight. Hold a pair of dumbbells with palms facing you.

Lift the dumbbells toward the ceiling while simultaneously turning the wrists so the palms point away from you.

- **Don't forget:** Avoid rounding your back.
- **You're working:** Your shoulders.

TIP!
- You can also perform this exercise while standing up.

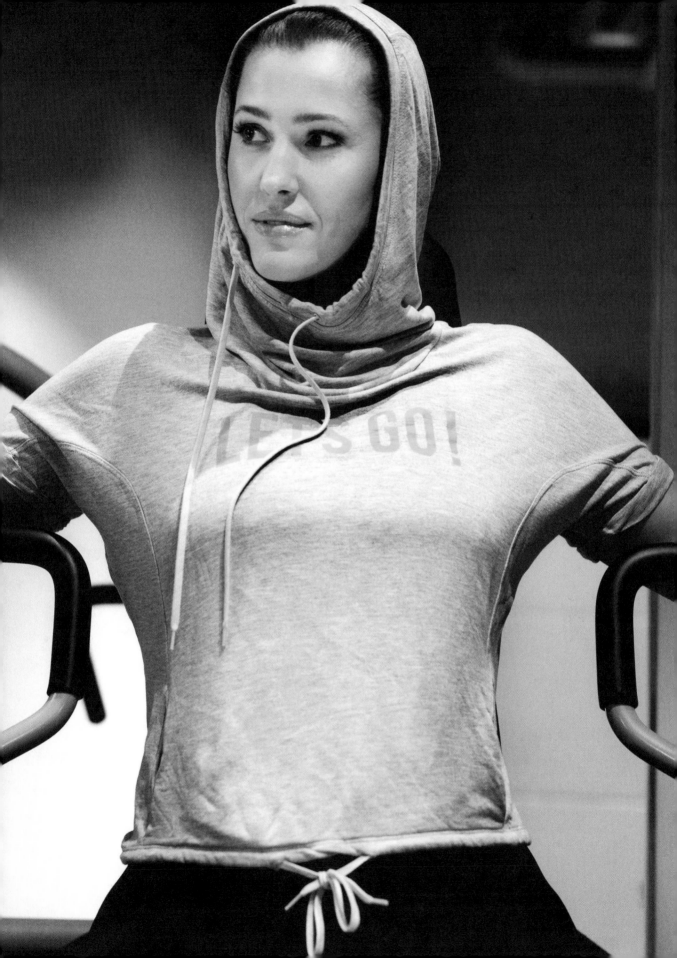

STEP 1—WORKOUT ROUTINE

ADJUST YOUR SETS AND REPETITIONS

If you are new to strength training, perform 2 sets of 15 repetitions, using light weights, for the first couple of weeks to let the joints and muscles become accustomed to the effort. Go up to 3 sets after three or four weeks, and then up to 4 sets after another three or four weeks, with the repetitions indicated below.

If you're an experienced lifter, start with 3 sets from the first week. Go up to 4 sets after about three weeks. Always focus on lifting heavier weights, keeping in mind the principles for strength training I've mentioned.

- **About midway through this step:** Begin lifting 6 to 8 reps instead of 5.
- **Before each workout:** Warm up, see page 76.
- **After each workout:** Stretches, see page 92.
- **Rest 1 minute between each set.**

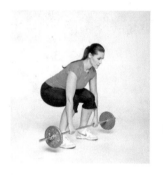

1. Barbell Dead Lift 1 P. 82
Set: **3** Repetitions: **5**

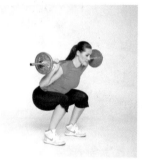

2. Squat with a Barbell P. 83
Set: **3** Repetitions: **5**

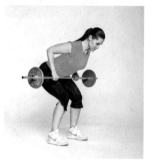

3. Bent Over Row P. 84
Set: **3** Repetitions: **5**

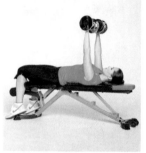

4. Dumbbell Bench Press P. 86
Set: **3** Repetitions: **5**

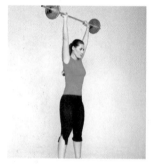

5. Military Shoulder Press P. 87
Set: **3** Repetitions: **5**

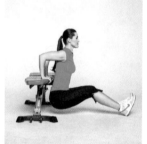

6. Dips P. 88
Set: **3** Repetitions: **15**

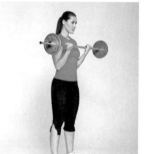

7. Barbell Biceps Curls P. 89
Set: **3** Repetitions: **5**

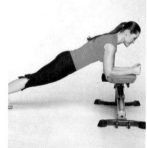

8. Bench Plank P. 90
Set: **3 x 1 minute**

If you're training in a gym, you can add the Pull Down and Rowing Machine after the Bent Over Row.

Pull Down P. 85
Set: **3** Repetitions: **5**

Rowing Machine P. 84
Set: **3** Repetitions: **5**

STEP 1—WEEKLY SCHEDULE

Monday:	Strength training
Tuesday:	Low intensity cardio
Wednesday:	Strength training
Thursday:	Low intensity cardio
Friday:	Strength training
Saturday:	Rest
Sunday:	Low intensity cardio

STEP 2—WORKOUT SCHEDULE

Note that the amount of sets and repetitions can vary, even though the exercises are the same in the steps. The fewer repetitions you do, the heavier the weights should be. Perform the French Press with dumbbells and the Dumbbell Bicep Curls in supersets, i.e., without rest between the exercises.

- **Before each workout:** Warm up, see page 76.
- **After each workout:** Stretches, see page 92.

MONDAY: **UPPER BODY**

- **Rest 1 minute between each set.**

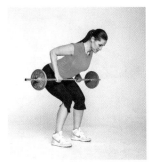

1. Bent Over Row   P. 84
Set: **4** Repetitions: **5**

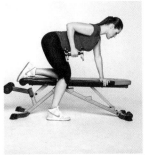

2. One Arm Row   P. 100
Set: **4** Repetitions: **6–8**

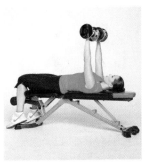

3. Dumbbell Bench Press   P. 86
Set: **4** Repetitions: **5**

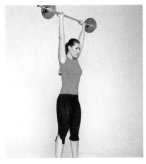

4. Military Shoulder Press   P. 87
Set: **4** Repetitions: **8–12**

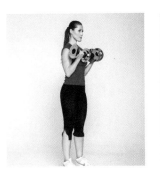

5. French Press with Dumbbells P. 101
Set: **4** Repetitions: **8–10**

6. Dumbbell Biceps Curls   P. 102
Set: **4** Repetitions: **8–10**

If you're working out in a gym, you can add the Pull Down after the One Arm Row.

Pull Down P. 85
Set: **4** Repetitions: **8**

STEP 2—WEEKLY SCHEDULE

Monday:	Upper body
Tuesday:	Lower body and core
Wednesday:	Low intensity cardio
Thursday:	Upper body
Friday:	Lower body and core
Saturday:	Rest
Sunday:	HIIT (alternate between the routines on page 98)

TUESDAY: **LOWER BODY + CORE**

• **Rest 1 minute between sets.**

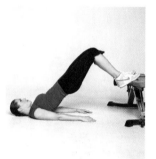

1. Glute Bridge　　P. 103
Set: **4** Repetitions: **15–20**

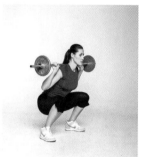

2. Barbell Deep Squat　　P. 104
Set: **4** Repetitions: **5**

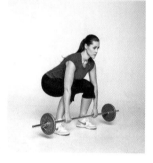

3. Dead Lift　　P. 105
Set: **4** Repetitions: **5**

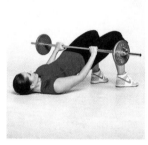

4. Hip Thrust　　P. 106
Set: **5** Repetitions: **8**

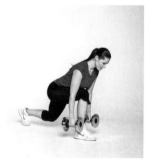

5. Incline Reverse Lunge　　P. 107
Set: **4** Repetitions: **15/leg**

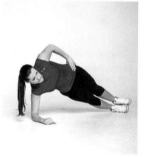

6. Side Hip Raises　　P. 108
Set: **4** Repetitions: **15–20/side**

THURSDAY: **UPPER BODY**

• **Rest 1 minute between sets.**

Perform the Incline Reverse Dumbbell Flies and the Seated Lateral Raise as a superset; do the same with the Dips and the Incline Dumbbells Bicep Curls. Rest 30 seconds between supersets.

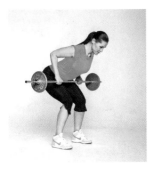

1. Bent Over Row P. 84
Set: **4** Repetitions: **8–12**

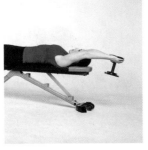

2. Pullover P. 109
Set: **4** Repetitions: **8–12**

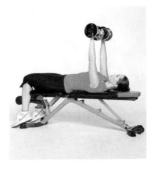

3. Dumbbell Bench Press P. 86
Set: **4** Repetitions: **8–12**

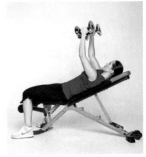

4. Incline Dumbbell Flies P. 110
Set: **4** Repetitions: **12–15**

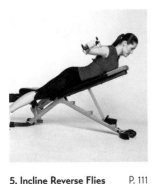

5. Incline Reverse Flies P. 111
Set: **4** Repetitions: **12–15**

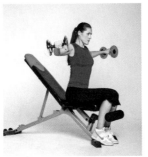

6. Seated Side Lateral Raise P. 112
Set: **4** Repetitions: **12–15**

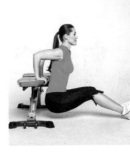

7. Dips P. 88
Set: **3** Repetitions: **to fatigue**

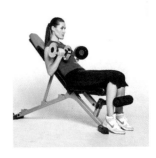

8. Incline Dumbbell Curls P. 113
Set: **3** Repetitions: **to fatigue**

If you're working out in a gym, add the Rowing Machine after the Bent Over Row.

Rowing Machine P. 84
Set: **4** Repetitions: **8**

FRIDAY: **UPPER BODY + CORE**

• **Rest 1 minute between sets.**

Do 4 sets of 8 to 12 repetitions for the Barbell Full Squat and the Dead Lift, immediately followed by set 5 of 20 repetitions at the same weight.

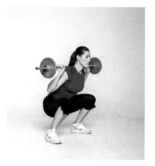

1. Barbell Deep Squat   P. 104
Set: **5** Repetitions: **8–12 + 1x20**

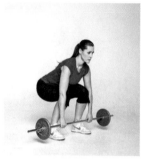

2. Dead Lift   P. 105
Set: **5** Repetitions: **8–12 + 1x20**

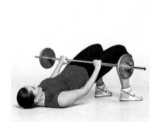

3. Hip Thrust   P. 106
Set: **5** Repetitions: **12–15**

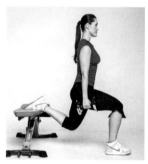

4. Bulgarian Split Squat   P. 114
Set: **5** Repetitions: **12–15/leg**

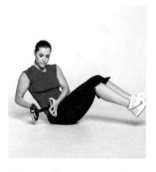

5. Russian Twist   P. 115
Set: **3** Repetitions: **to fatigue**

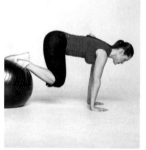

6. Stability Ball Knee Tuck-In P. 116
Set: **3** Repetitions: **to fatigue**

STEP 3—WORKOUT ROUTINES

- **Before each workout:** Warm up, see page 76.
- **After each workout:** Stretches, see page 92.

MONDAY: LOWER BODY

- **Rest 1 minute between each set.**

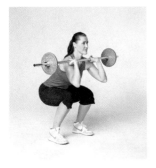

1. Front Squat   P. 122
Set: **5** Repetitions: **6–8**

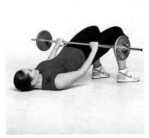

2. Hip Thrust   P. 106
Set: **5** Repetitions: **8**

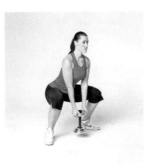

3. Wide-Stance Dumbbell Squat   P. 123
Set: **5** Repetitions: **15**

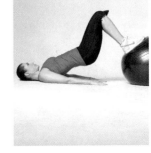

4. Stability Ball Hip Roll   P. 124
Set: **4** Repetitions: **15–20**

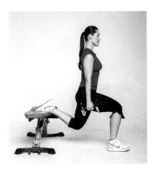

5. Bulgarian Split Squat   P. 114
Set: **5** Repetitions: **6–8/leg**

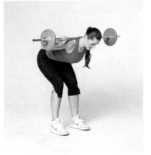

6. Good Mornings   P. 125
Set: **5** Repetitions: **15–20**

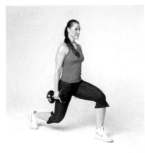

7. Walking Lunge with Dumbbells   P. 126
Set: **5** Repetitions: **10/leg**

STEP 3—WEEKLY SCHEDULE

Monday:	Lower body
Tuesday:	Low intensity cardio, 45 minutes
Wednesday:	Metabolic circuit training
Thursday:	HIIT 1 workout, with 30 minutes of low intensity cardio
Friday:	Upper body
Saturday:	Rest
Sunday:	HIIT 2 workout, with 30 minutes low intensity cardio

WEDNESDAY: **METABOLIC CIRCUIT TRAINING**

Alternate between 8 and 15 repetitions every second week in this circuit. Every week you'll use heavier weights and perform 8 repetitions, and every alternate week you'll use lighter weights and do 15 repetitions. In Step Ups with Dumbbells, you'll do 8 or 15 repetitions for each leg. Go through the exercises without resting in between, and don't rest until after the Stability Ball Hip Raise. Then, take a 2-minute rest.

In the first weeks you can do the workout with 4 sets; after three weeks you can increase the sets to 5; after another three weeks bump it up to 6 sets.

• **Rest 1 minute between each set**

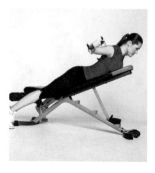
1. Incline Reverse Flies   P. 111

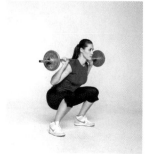
2. Barbell Deep Squat   P. 104

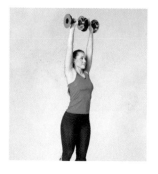
3. Push Press with Dumbbells   P. 127

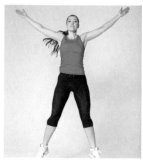
4. Jumping Jacks   P. 128

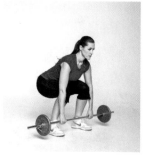
5. Dead Lift   P. 105

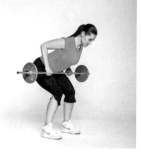
6. Bent Over Row   P. 84

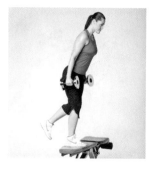
7. Step Ups with Dumbbells   P. 129

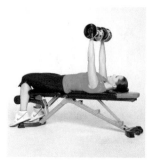
8. Dumbbell Bench Press   P. 86

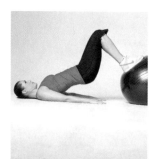
9. Stability Ball Hip Roll   P. 124

FRIDAY: **UPPER BODY**

• **Rest 1 minute between sets.**

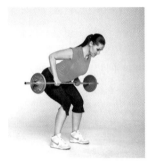

1. Bent Over Row   P. 84
Set: **4** Repetitions: **6–8**

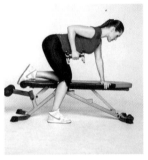

2. One Arm Row   P. 100
Set: **4** Repetitions: **6–8/arm**

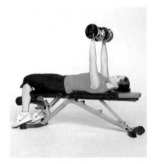

3. Dumbbell Bench Press   P. 86
Set: **4** Repetitions: **6–8**

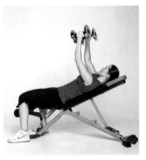

4. Incline Dumbbell Flies   P. 110
Set: **4** Repetitions: **12–15**

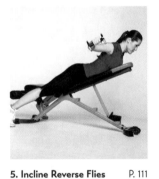

5. Incline Reverse Flies   P. 111
Set: **4** Repetitions: **12–15**

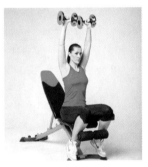

6. Arnold Press   P. 130
Set: **4** Repetitions: **12–15**

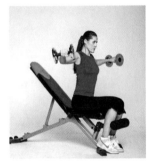

7. Seated Side Lateral Raise   P. 112
Set: **4** Repetitions: **12–15**

If you work out in a gym, start with the Pull Down and the Rowing Machine.

Pull Down   P. 85
Set: **4** Repetitions: **8**

Rowing Machine   P. 84
Set: **4** Repetitions: **8**

FINAL WORDS

First of all: Huge congratulations are in order for persevering! I really hope that you have achieved what you set out to do and that you feel stronger and more energetic. Now that you've come to the end of this book, what are you going to do next? How are you going to work out? How are you going to eat?

Nowadays, numerous books, articles, and other media focus on weight loss, workouts, diets, lowering cholesterol, and getting rid of stress in the shortest amount of time possible. But what do you do once you've gotten there? Very little emphasis is placed on how to maintain your gains and achieve what everyone is after—balance. It's not unusual that many put weight back on after a while because they don't know how to keep things going once they've reached their goal. Balance means continuing to eat high quality foods and working out; you have not earned a break. No, this is when the real challenge begins: to put into daily practice everything you've learned, perhaps without so much measuring and weighing.

Hopefully you're pleased with your weight and have found a way to nourish yourself satisfactorily. If you seek further guidance, calculate your current BMR, continue keeping a food journal, and remember the importance of calorie allotment.

While all my workouts can be incorporated into your future training, I feel that the routines in step 2 are especially well suited for continued exercise. If you wish to build more muscle mass, perform the book's steps over again (but don't forget to adjust your diet for each step and your new goals). If you want to challenge yourself even further, I'd be more than happy to encourage you to follow me and my training plans online at www.mammafitness.se (in Swedish).

Trust yourself. Are you hungry? Eat more. Are you full? Then stop eating. Are you exhausted? If you feel tired, exhausted, or unmotivated, take a week's break from your workouts (not from a proper diet, however!). This doesn't mean you shouldn't move; instead, engage in some relaxing, low intensity cardio workouts. What I'm saying is that you should listen to your body. Health is not measured in workouts or the number of calories you consume but in how you feel and your quality of life.

Somewhere along the line you will reach the point where you'll make peace with yourself and choose to work out to maintain what you have accomplished. Eating without guilt, feeling motivated by your progress, viewing your health as a priority, and finding your base level (the minimum amount of exercise you need to do on a weekly basis to stay in shape) won't be accomplished overnight. To that I say: What's the rush? You are investing in your new lifestyle.

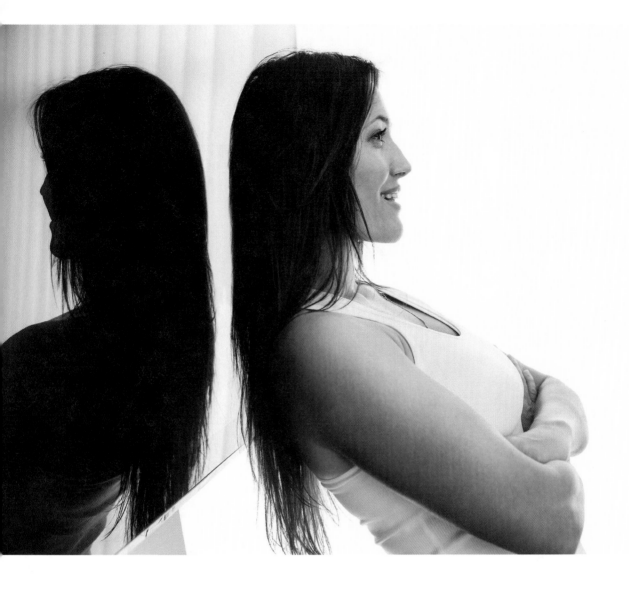

THANK YOU!

A huge thanks to all my clients and to all of you who follow me on social media! Thank you for putting your trust in me and for not giving up.
Thank you Malin Forslund, our nutritionist at MammaFitness, for checking the accuracy of the nutritional calculations.
Thank you to my husband, for all his support during this project.
Thank you to Linnéa von Zweigbergk and Kerstin Bergfors, for their continued confidence in me.
Thank you to Andreas Lundberg for his pictures—I won't forget our sessions. His imagination is inspirational!
Thank you to Anders Timrén, for a great layout.

WORKOUT LOG

DATE ....

EXERCISE	SET	REPETITION	LBS/KG

REFLECTIONS ON WORKOUT:

FOOD JOURNAL

DATE ....

MEAL	RECIPE/INGREDIENTS	AMOUNT	KCAL
		TOTAL:	

COMMENTARY:

REFERENCES

Ivey, FM, et al (2000): "Effects of age, gender, and myostatin genotype on the hypertrophic response to heavy resistance strength training." *The Journals of Gerontology, Series A: Biological Sciences and Medical Sciences*, vol. 55, no.11.

Martell GF, et al (2006): "Age and sex affect human muscle fibre adaptations to heavy-resistance strength training." *Experimental Physiology*, vol. 91, no.2.

Staron RS, et al (1990): "Muscle hypertrophy and fast fibre type conversions in heavy resistance-trained women." *European Journal of Applied Physiology and Occupational Physiology*, vol. 60.

Annerstedt, C, and Gjerset, A (1997): *Idrottens träningslära* (SISU Idrottsböcker).

Baechle, TR, and Earle, RW (2000): *Essentials of Strength Training and Conditioning.* (Human Kinetics).

Carlstedts, J (1997): *Styrketräning för att bli snabb, stark eller uthållig.* (SISU Idrottsböcker).

Kang, J (2008): *Bioenergetics Primer for Exercise Science.* (Human Kinetics).

Maughan, RJ (2000): *Nutrition in Sport*, vol. 7 *of The Encyclopaedia of Sports Nutrition* (Blackwell).

Runge, MS, and Patterson, C (2006) *Principles of Molecular Medicine* (Humana Press).

Wolinsky, I, and Driskell, JA (2008): *Sports Nutrition: Energy Metabolism and Exercise* (CRC Press).

National Research Council (2005): "Dietary Reference Intakes for Energy, Carbohydrate, Fiber, Fat, Fatty Acids, Cholesterol, Protein, and Amino Acids"(The National Academies Press).

Zawadzki, KM, Yaspelkis III, BB, and Ivy, JL (1992): "Carbohydrate-protein complex increases the rate of muscle glycogen storage after exercise." *Journal of Applied Physiology*, vol. 72, no. 5.

Jentjens, RL, et al (2001): "Addition of protein and amino acids to carbohydrates does not exhance postexercise muscle glycogen synthesis." *Journal of Applied Physiology*, vol. 91, no. 2.

Juul, A, and Jorgensen, JOL (2000): *Growth Hormone in Adults: Physiological and Clinical Aspects* (Cambridge University Press).

Plowman, SA, Smith, DL (2007): *Exercise Physiology for Health, Fitness, and Performance* (LWW).